ALTERNATIVE TREATMENTS FOR ANIMALS

A Guide to Naturally Healing Cats, Dogs, Horses, and More for Owners and Caregivers

Lisa Preston

Foreword by RACE FOSTER, DVM

Skyhorse Publishing

Copyright © 2020 by Lisa Preston

All Rights Reserved. No part of this book may be reproduced in any manner without the express written consent of the publisher, except in the case of brief excerpts in critical reviews or articles. All inquiries should be addressed to Skyhorse Publishing, 307 West 36th Street, 11th Floor, New York, NY 10018.

Skyhorse Publishing books may be purchased in bulk at special discounts for sales promotion, corporate gifts, fund-raising, or educational purposes. Special editions can also be created to specifications. For details, contact the Special Sales Department, Skyhorse Publishing, 307 West 36th Street, 11th Floor, New York, NY 10018 or info@skyhorsepublishing.com.

Skyhorse® and Skyhorse Publishing® are registered trademarks of Skyhorse Publishing, Inc.®, a Delaware corporation.

www.skyhorsepublishing.com

10 9 8 7 6 5 4 3 2 1

Library of Congress Cataloging-in-Publication Data is available on file.

Cover design by Kai Texel
Cover photos by gettyimages

Print ISBN: 978-1-5107-5142-2
Ebook ISBN: 978-1-62636-604-6

Printed in China

I solemnly swear to use my scientific knowledge and
skills . . . for the protection of animal health.
—**The Veterinarian's Oath**

The most beautiful and most profound experience
is the sensation of the mystical. It is the sower
of all true science.
—**Albert Einstein**

Contents

Foreword

BY RACE FOSTER, DVM

KEEPING ANIMALS HEALTHY has evolved into a profession called veterinary medicine. Historically, those who knew the most about animals were the chosen ones to provide advice. In this country, General George Washington recognized the need for animal health and helped to elevate the farriers because of their hands-on approach to and knowledge of animals. It was the farrier that oftentimes provided "veterinary care."

In the mid- and late 1800s came the development of the great teaching institutions, and veterinary medicine became a professional degree. A degree earned gave the graduate the right to practice veterinary medicine and devise a living from keeping animals healthy.

For over one hundred years, veterinary science has attempted to unravel the secrets of disease prevention and treatment. Success has been overwhelming; but much remains to be discovered, and the quest for full answers will be eternal.

The modern-day veterinary practitioners are armed with a huge base of scientific data to support their understanding of animal disease processes. Additionally, modern medicine has provided us with a wide array of drugs and medications to support our treatments.

Once a disease or disorder is recognized, it may or may not be treatable. Usually we think of treatments as involving manufactured drugs; some good, some potentially bad. The educated veterinarian of today also recognizes the potential use of alternative therapies, most described in the text of this book.

Alternative treatments are real and can be extremely beneficial. Remember that before modern science, alternative treatments were all that was available, and there is no argument from me that their benefits have withstood the test of time. Outside of modern science, maybe, but beneficial.

In reviewing the contents of this book, I realized how much I need to learn. I cannot be a good and credible veterinarian if I am passive to the possibilities that alternative treatments provide. In reading this book, I have become a better veterinarian, and the animal kingdom will be better for it. Every veterinary teaching institution, veterinarian, and pet owner should similarly become informed. Reading the following pages will help them accomplish that.

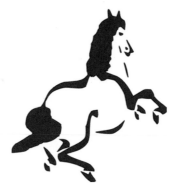

Introduction to the New Edition

WHEN MY PUBLISHER asked for an updated edition of *Natural Healing for Cats, Dogs, Horses and Other Animals*, I was delighted. More products, more practitioners, more research, and critical thinking all begged for inclusion.

Terrific well-controlled studies have made it possible to explore how science is needed to shed light on well-accepted beliefs that can turn out to be dead wrong. Cannabis products are now entering the realm of the legal in many locations. In the first edition, I hadn't said enough about essential oils. EndoTapping has offered interesting results. I wanted to compare VitaFlex and RainDrop technique. Fine distinctions between some manual therapies means that there are more choices than ever to help heal animals. New studies showed new results in pheromone therapy. Devices were developed to enable double-blind testing of acupuncture. Stem cell therapies are promising, yet sales have outpaced the science, which means animal owners must become better informed about the products and services they consider for their pets.

Yes, the world of alternative therapies for animals has only expanded, and it has been a fascinating journey bringing my readers this new edition of *Natural Healing for Cats, Dogs, Horses and Other Animals*. Enjoy, and do keep in touch. I love to engage with readers, no matter whether they are for or against alternative treatments.

—Lisa Preston

www.lisapreston.com

PART 1

CRITICAL THINKING

Orientation: Before You Explore

CONTROVERSY ABOUNDS IN the field of alternative treatments, even regarding the very terms used to describe the collective array of therapies available. Some people rightly point out that even the term *alternative treatment* is problematic because conventional treatment frequently offers multiple proven options—alternatives—for a specific medical condition. This argument treads around the reality: We all know we are talking about treatments that are generally an alternative to conventional medicine. But things get murkier still. Some refer to *complementary and alternative medicine (CAM)* as a set of options or adjuncts to conventional modern medicine. Complementary or *integrative medicine* seeks to combine alternatives with conventional medicine. By integrating alternatives with conventional care, proponents hope to achieve the best of both worlds. Therapies considered in place of standard medical practice are necessarily nonstandard treatments, because if they were standard conventional care, then they could not be labeled alternatives.

The strictest conventional medical view is that alternative treatments, as the term is commonly understood, are unproven, therefore ineffective and a waste of time and money at best, quackery and fraud at worst. But, more and more, people are making the dogleg turn away from conventional medicine and toward alternative options for care. And more and more, modern medicine must take these alternatives seriously. Thus, if a treatment is called alternative, then to what is it an alternative? An alternative to standard conventional care? Why would anyone choose a nonstandard treatment that is not accepted by the best clinicians, the best universities? This question will be explored even before we examine the multitude of treatments now available for animals, but we'll first agree to simply call them alternatives and not further belabor the term.

Natural Healing for Cats, Dogs, Horses, and Other Animals is an overview of nontraditional therapies and treatments available for animals. It examines dozens of choices without promoting any one particular method. It compares the advantages and disadvantages of these alternative treatments and then offers specific advice on what to look for and what to avoid in choosing a practitioner.

Many books are available to guide a layperson through some aspect of alternative treatment, for example a book focusing on herbal remedies or aromatherapy. Most of these books tend to approach the therapy from an advocate's position without necessarily demanding to know: Does it work? This is a question that must be asked, and the answer is generally tenuous and anecdotal, avoiding strict science. Some advocates openly discourage questioning, or cannot answer the hard questions. Other guides reject all alternative therapies—an approach that, when rendered by a member of conventional mainstream medicine, can appear to be turf guarding.

It's good to ask questions, indeed to explore alternative treatments with skepticism. Let's try for a neutral approach, examining both the advocates' and the detractors' views of each treatment. If we do less than this, we haven't really examined all treatment options.

There are dozens of veterinary colleges in the United States, Canada, Australia, and the United Kingdom. While some of these veterinary programs engage some alternative therapies, it is fair to say the general scientific community of established veterinarians does not wholly embrace all alternative treatments examined in this book.

Are the alternative treatments discussed here just New Age phenomena? No. In fact, many alternatives predate modern medicine. Further, one would hesitate to categorically term alternatives to conventional veterinary treatment as not having a tradition behind them, even though they are thought of by some as nontraditional treatments. For example, traditional Chinese medicine (often referred to as TCM), including veterinary care, is often touted to have been followed for several millennia. Of course, herbal remedies have a longer history than does modern medicine. Neanderthals used comfrey and other botanical medicines. Ayurveda, an ancient folk medicine from the Indian subcontinent, is still practiced today.

However, learning should not entail a battle between Eastern and Western medicine. While some therapies discussed in these pages would be accurately classified under the realm of Eastern medicine (including acupuncture, acupressure, ayurveda, reiki, and numbers of herbal remedies), some treatments were founded in Europe, such as homeopathy and naturopathy, while reflexology is thought by some to have come from ancient Egypt. Other treatments, such as chiropractic and NAET (Nambudripad Allergy Elimination Technique) came from North America.

So what alternative treatments are available for our animals? The list is staggering and sometimes overlapping.

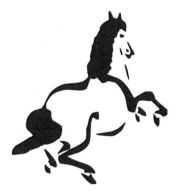

List of Alternative Treatments

CHIROPRACTORS, HOMEOPATHS, naturopaths, holistic veterinarians, and other practitioners of alternative treatments for animals may employ any of the following alternative treatments and diagnostic methods. (Therapies known by more than one name are also listed here by those synonyms.)

Acupressure	Chakra Adjustment
Acupuncture	Chelation Therapy
Alpha-Stim	Chi/Ji/Ki/Qi Adjustment
Anma	Chiropractic
Apitherapy	Chromotherapy
Aquapuncture	Cold Laser
Aquatic Massage Therapy (AMT)	Colloidal Minerals
Aromatherapy	Colloidal Silver
Astrology	Color Therapy
Augmentation Therapy	Craniosacral Therapy
Aura Adjustment	Crystal Healing
Aural Photography	Cupping
Auriculotherapy	Dark Field Microscopy (DFM)
Ayurveda	Diatomaceous Earth
Bach Flower Remedies	Deep Connective Tissue Massage
Biochemic Tissue Salts	Deep Muscle Therapy
Bioplasma	Detoxification Therapy
Botanicals	Dowsing
Bowen Technique	Effleurage
Cannabis Products	Electroacupuncture
Cell Salts	Electrodermal Testing
Cell Therapy	Electromagnetic Therapy

Electrophoresis

Endotapping

Energy Emission Analysis (EEA)

Essential Oils

Extracorporeal Shock Wave
    Therapy (ESWT)

Fascial Manipulation

Feng Shui

Flower Essences

Functional Medicine

Galvanic Skin Response Scanning

Gemmotherapy

Glandular Therapy

Gold Beads

Hair Analysis

Hair Mineral Analysis (HMA)

Harmonic Medicine

Heliotherapy

Hemp Oil

Herbalism

Homeopathy

Homotoxicology

Hydrotherapy

Hyperbaric Oxygen Treatment
    (HBOT)

Hypnosis

Immuno-Augmentive Therapy

Infrasound

Infratonic Therapy

Integrative Manual Therapy (IMT)

Intrinsic Data Field Analysis

Iontophoresis

Iridology

Kinergetics

Kinesiology

Kirlian Assessment

Larval Therapy

Laser Therapy

Limbic Massage

Live Blood Analysis

Live Cell Therapy

Lomilomi

Low Energy Photon Therapy
    (LEPT)

Low-Level Laser Therapy (LLLT)

Maggot Therapy

Magnetic Therapy

Manual Lymph Drain (MLD)

Massage

Medicinal Mushrooms

Megavitamin Therapy

Mesenchymal Stromal Cells

Mesotherapy

Microcurrent/Microamperage
    Electrical Neuromuscular
    Stimulation (MENS)

Moxibustion

Muscle Response Testing

Myofascial Release

Nambudripad's Allergy
    Elimination Technique
    (NAET)

Naturopathy

Neural Therapy

Neuromuscular Electrical
    Stimulation (NMES)

Newcastle Treatment

Nosodes

Nutraceuticals

Nutrigenomics

Nutrition Therapy

Orthomolecular Medicine

Osteopathy

Ozone Therapy

Pendulum Assessment

Petrissage

Pheromone Therapy

Photonic Therapy

Platelet-Rich Plasma (PRP)

Polyfrequency Spectrum Testing

Polysan

Pressure Garments

Prolotherapy

Pulsed/Pulsating
   Electromagnetic Field
   Therapy (PEMF)

Psychic Analysis/Communication

Psychosomatic Energetics

Qigong

Qxci Quantum Healing

Radionics

RainDrop Technique

ReBa Testing

Reflexology

Regenerative Medicine

Reiki

Rolfing

Saliva Testing

Sanum Remedies

Sclerotherapy

Segmental Therapy

Self-Controlling Energo
   Neuro Adaptive Regulation
   (SCENAR)

Shiatsu

Sonic Therapy

Sonography

Stem Cells

BELOW: Choices abound in alternative care. Making the best decision for an animal requires careful consideration.

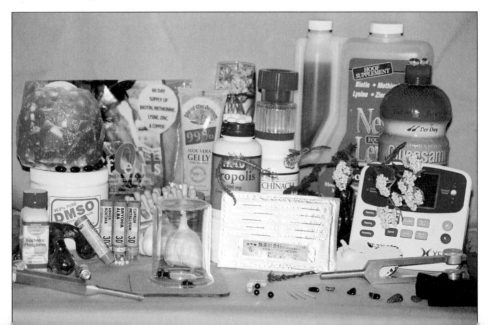

Tai Ji

Therapeutic Touch

Thought Field Therapy (TFT)

Ting Point Therapy

Tissue Salts

Tongue-Pulse Diagnosis

Traditional Chinese Medicine/
   Traditional Chinese
   Veterinary Medicine (TCM/
   TCVM)

Transcutaneous Electrical
   Neuromuscular Stimulation
   (TENS)

Trigger Point Therapy

Ttouch

Tui Na

Tuning Fork Therapy

Ultrasonography

Veterinary Orthopedic
   Manipulation (VOM)

Vibrational Therapy

Vita Flex

Water (Acidified, Activated,
   Alkalinized, Clustered,
   Energized, Hexagonal,
   Inducted, Ionized, Live,
   Oxygenated, Pentagonal,
   Structured)

Watsu

Zero Balancing

Do You Have to Be a Believer? The Skeptics' Story

A couple's dog scraped his hind legs jumping a fence. The wounds did not seem bad enough to require a trip to the veterinarian, so they gently cleaned the abrasions and then simply left them alone. After a few days, when the dog licked the wounds excessively, they carefully bandaged his legs.

They thought it was a minor problem. However, the dog licked the bandages. Soon, he chewed the bandages off and went back to licking the scrapes. A month passed during which they tried more bandages with bad-tasting sprays on them. Still, the dog licked his bandages off and pestered the wounds incessantly. Their veterinarian examined the dog, noted the very poor healing of simple scrapes, and recommended an Elizabethan collar.

"An eighty-pound dog can push over a lot of stuff walking around the house with a stiff plastic collar strapped around his neck, and he can get pretty pouty as well," the man said. They didn't want to disrupt their household or make their dog unhappy; they just wanted him to let his legs heal.

The veterinarian identified the problem as canine lick granuloma. She wanted to try acupuncture and further wanted to show the couple how to do it. They were skeptical but didn't have a better reason not to try it other than, well, they just didn't believe in it. One of the owners asked the vet how acupuncture worked.

"I don't know," the vet said. And she told them that it doesn't always work but she persuaded the clients to give it a try.

So they learned to put tiny needles near the scrapes.

"Our dog didn't seem to mind at all," the woman said, "but then this was a dog who never cared about shots either. We left the needles in for ten minutes or so, like the vet said to do. We were to do this home acupuncture treatment several times a week. In less than a week however, something amazing happened. He quit licking the scrapes, and real healing finally began. We wished we'd tried acupuncture weeks and weeks earlier."

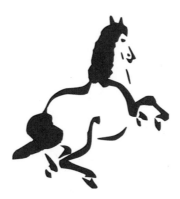

The Big Boom in Alternative Treatments

WHY IS THERE such an apparent increase in alternative treatment and holistic care?

An abundance of *anecdotal evidence*—a funny term for stories that are not actual evidence but rather are stories from people like the couple above who report solving their dog's wound-licking through acupuncture—increases the appeal of alternatives. Perhaps less admirable reasons include iconoclasm and a blanket rejection of modern medicine. Ascetics and minimalists may naturally turn to alternative care as a primary choice.

Another factor giving rise to the burgeoning interest in alternative treatments may be related to an increased population naturally leading to an increased use of every option. Also, globalization and rapid communication via the Internet and other modalities have dramatically sped the transfer of knowledge and ideas, making more people aware of the range of alternatives available. Perhaps there is more open-mindedness now than ever before, and certainly, people want to be smart consumers. We want to know what's wrong, and we want to understand our choices when deciding what to do about a problem.

But we don't want to be duped.

Oversight for the alternative treatment side of animal health is variable. In the United States, industry regulation comes from—and is missed by—overlapping and conflicting interests. The U.S. Food and Drug Administration's Center for Veterinary Medicine regulates food additives, drugs, and devices that are administered to animals, with the exception of vaccines (which are regulated by the U.S. Department of Agriculture's Center for Veterinary Biologics), but neither Center handles the vast alternative supplements administered by the various alternative practitioners for animals. The National Animal Supplement Council is a trade organization of companies that promote supplements for animals, but no one organization studies whether any of these alternatives have any efficacy.

Human and animal physiology have so much in common that answers and education sought for one species may initially be found in reviewing treatment testing on another species. It is crucial to remember, however, that species are not interchangeable, and efficacy must eventually be demonstrated on the animal species being treated. For example, dogs can process certain artificial sweeteners—alcohol sugars—that humans cannot, and thus can become critically hyperglycemic on a product that gives no digestible sugar or calories to a human. The meat-eating cat and the grass-eating horse have very different nutritional and supplementation needs, behaviors (one being a predator and the other being a prey animal) and rest requirements (one happily sleeping about twenty hours a day while the other stays awake for the same number of hours). So when searching for information on a problem or a possible treatment, first look broadly, but then narrow the examination to the same kind of animal in the same circumstances. The big boom has put a great deal of information out for the consumer, but we have to be smart consumers of that information.

In broad study of the alternatives, tremendous recognition and effort has been made. In 1991, Congress funded the Office of Alternative Medicine and, in 1998, this office was elevated to a National Institutes of Health Office. By 1999, the Office became the National Center for Complementary and Alternative Medicine. Clearly, the big boom in alternative treatments has caused a complementary boom in research and information.

What else has provoked the interest? There is an understandable desire to avoid side effects and complications from strong medications. Some people may turn to alternative therapies with a hope of keeping costs down. Wanting to have explored every possibility in caring for a beloved pet is a motivating factor for some people who try nontraditional therapies. We want to do all that can be done. Also, many people have an undeniable urge for natural care and treatment.

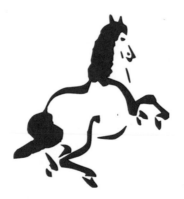

Know What Is Natural and What Is Nonsense

ISN'T NATURE JUST naturally more natural, and isn't that a Good Thing?

First, we have to define our terms. What is *natural*? And let's consider not just what natural means but also why we think it's wonderful. It certainly sounds healthy, but then, strictly speaking, many diseases can be regarded as perfectly natural, as are many poisons. Eventual death is certainly natural. Some might think of any prescription as unnatural, and some might find many of the alternative treatments explored here unnatural. Because we can all define the word differently, we must ask the practitioner who advocates *natural care* what he or she means by the term.

Some people portray pharmaceutical companies as akin to a secret cabal dominating health care. These people might eschew all commercial drug therapies prescribed by modern veterinarians. A more moderate approach accepts the need for serious medication in serious situations but wants to avoid strong chemicals and strong side effects whenever reasonable.

Remember, a rejection of all things synthetic demands rejecting a simple vitamin C tablet. Some all-natural proponents decry pet diets that are widely deemed acceptable by the best veterinarians at the best universities. Many herbs recommended by alternative treatment practitioners are toxic. It is an ironic tragedy that a person may accidentally harm an animal while trying to give it natural, alternative treatment. Caring for an animal should not be a matter of guesswork or amateurism, and making smart choices takes considerable effort. The U.S. Food and Drug Administration's GRAS list—a published list of substances Generally Recognized as Safe—will not help someone trying to decide if an unlisted substance is safe to try. And not every veterinarian will be enthused about a client wanting more information that could result in consumers taking business elsewhere. Separating the safe from the dangerous or silly is largely left to the individual.

Nonsensical claims of healing that fly in the face of all logic abound, and what works for one animal might not work for another. If a practitioner says he can adjust your dog's chi, correct his energy along proper meridians, or has a tonic that can treat a wide array of completely unrelated problems, shouldn't we ask for proof? And what should we accept as proof?

BELOW: **Chromotherapy, heliotherapy, chakra adjustment. Can a blue light bath soothe this cat?**

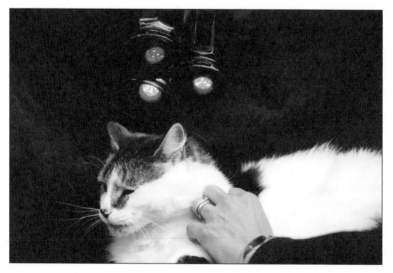

Science, Proof, and Placebos

THERE IS A spectrum along which all treatments, both conventional and alternative, fall. At one end would be widely accepted conventional modern medicine, including surgery and pharmaceutical intervention, generally backed by numerous studies. At the other end of the spectrum would be highly mystical processes or actions that have never been broadly documented as successful in healing.

Modern medicine was, of course, preceded by folk traditions, herbal treatments, and superstitions. Hippocrates, born around 460 BC, is often considered to be the father of Western medicine. He established the rule of doing no further harm and the need to perform a detailed physical examination of the patient. However, anatomy and physiology were not understood for many, many more centuries. Not having a modern understanding of the body's form and function, conjecture by early peoples created all manner of myths and hypotheses to fill the void.

Ancient Greeks believed there were four *humors* (black bile, yellow bile, blood, and phlegm), and they linked each of these fluids to one of the following characteristics, which they deemed essential: warm, cool, dry, and wet. They further linked personality types and seasons to each humor, as well as what they considered the four elements: earth, air, fire, and water. Believing in their concept of these four humors, and believing humoral imbalance to be responsible for illnesses, led to bloodletting and purging as primitive medical treatments. Paralleled in India and China, these ancient Greek concepts lasted for many, many centuries. Western medicine only slowly became modern science, with a careful method of inquiry, starting in the last few hundred years and accelerating in progress rapidly in the last century.

Vitalism, the belief that vital forces controlled life, was entrenched in ancient times. Beliefs in prana, chakra, aura, or chi are examples of vitalism, with modern proponents viewing the concept of an animal's vital life force as distinct from physical and chemical processes understood in modern physiology. Like vitalism, many folk cures have been preserved, with some of these resurfacing as alternative treatments in modern times. The difficulty lies in intelligently examining the vast alternatives with an open mind.

One guide to alternative treatments completely rejects nearly every nonconventional therapy available. Dozens of books on alternative therapies and so-called natural pet care point to real case studies—anecdotes—in an attempt to prove their efficacy, but genuine proof is something else entirely.

Within these lay guides, there is a startling lack of information on physical examination and assessment. A foundation of conventional medicine is its emphasis on patient assessment. No one who is not competent at assessing animals should ever assess an animal without proper guidance or training. A listless animal at rest with a weak, rapid pulse has a very different problem from a listless animal at rest with a strong heartbeat at an appropriately moderate tempo—and pulse is just one sign used in making a thorough physical assessment of a patient.

While good patient-assessment skills should be found among conventional and alternative practitioners, there are certainly charlatans who lack this basic knowledge. Alternative treatments do not exist on their own. They need practitioners to provide them. It is reasonable to ask these practitioners to defend their knowledge, their success, and their familiarity with both traditional therapy and their recommended nontraditional treatment. They should also reveal any potential conflict of interest. Someone who sells a specific herb preparation, for example, is not in the best position to claim that it is the best remedy for any particular ailment.

Science

Modern bioscience will embrace and swallow alternative methods that are proven to work. In effect, an alternative treatment can graduate to conventional medicine, because once a modality is well proven, it is no longer alternative—it's mainstream.

To reasonably identify a specific remedy as effective for a specific ailment, science turns to empirical, evidence-based medicine. Veterinary education follows this trend. The largest mainstream veterinary group in North America is the American Veterinary Medical Association (AVMA). AVMA's guidelines on complementary and alternative medicine identify a need for all treatments to meet the scientific standards equivalent to those of mainstream medicine.

Standard scientific testing includes: studies over as large a sample population as possible (large sample); a random selection in which some of the population are given the treatment and some are given only inert treatment (randomization); a placebo (control); both the subject population and the examiners not knowing until after the treatment course which patients received the placebo and which received the study treatment (double-blind); releasing the study design and results to professional colleagues for independent examination (peer review); and reproducible results—that is, a repeated study should make a similar finding.

In poorly controlled studies, self-serving bias occurs when unexplained positive consequences are attributed to a treatment without causation necessarily being proven. Other errors of attribution, spurious relationships, and counterfactual claims muddy attempts to prove alternatives.

Modern science further relies on contemporary teachings of anatomy and physiology, even when attempting to consider ideas outside the realm of what they believe to be true. Intangible concepts of life forces simply cannot fit under the scientific realm.

The Problem of Proof

Although good scientific studies of treatments are peer-reviewed, double-blind, randomized, reproducible, controlled, and conducted over large samples, they still have difficulty pointing to absolute cause and effect because living beings are so complex and there are many factors that can affect an animal and a treatment. There tends to be a natural waxing and waning of many illnesses, with many people seeking help only when things are at their worst. The horse's lameness, the cat's lethargy, the dog being off his feed—all might have improved without the visit to the veterinarian if the animal's condition naturally improved. In many cases, there is no way of knowing absolutely if improvement is due to the treatment, the animal, or the disease process winding down.

Anecdotes and testimonials, such as that of the couple who tried acupuncture to treat their dog's excessive licking, are not proof of a treatment's efficacy.

Cognitive bias in the form of subject-expectancy effect occurs when the patient expects a certain effect from a treatment. While animals may not be susceptible to this, the people who care for them are; and it is us, the animal lovers, who experience the observer-expectancy effect and may report improvement that does not exist. Regression to the mean and cognitive dissonance may also be misinterpreted as resulting from a treatment under study.

Animals are both better and worse subjects than people for evaluating a treatment. People can tell us how they feel. Animals exhibit signs, symptoms, and behavior without speech. People lie, both intentionally and unintentionally. They might misstate how long their dog is left unattended or how much he is exercised, because they mean to do better by the animal in the future and are adjusting their answer to what they plan on doing, not what they are actually doing. They might have missed observing the dog vomiting and report that he is no longer vomiting. Some animals are incredibly stoic, and some superficially appear to have the same countenance whether they are in pain or simply resting.

Most evaluations of animals have a significant subjective factor, however. For example, while a vital sign such as pulse or temperature is an absolute number, external factors influence vital signs. A person who wants her animal to feel better and is anxiously looking for signs of improvement may report improvement where none concretely exists. This can be a matter of the placebo response in reporting or observer-expectancy. Also, while some people erroneously report that there is no such thing as an actual placebo response among animals, the placebo effect has been demonstrated in some instances. Some animals respond to a simple saline injection where others are given a drug. In humans, this is termed the subject-expectancy.

Placebos

In numerous tests of both traditional and nontraditional treatments, patients who were not actually given the treatment got better. This improvement may be called the placebo response, and some people believe it occurs in animals as well as in humans, although the effect tends to be less pronounced in animals (and children).

After this placebo response became known among physicians, the undisclosed administration of placebos for various complaints began. The obvious ethical problem of this kind of placebo administration helped diminish intentional placebo prescriptions. However, the placebo response remains one quick explanation when someone dismisses observed improvement in an animal who is given alternative treatment.

Diseases and disorders run their natural course, letting animal health improve. This is another common explanation from naysayers regarding presumed benefit from an alternative. But how can we conclusively determine what makes an animal get better?

Lurking variables confound test results, which can then be misinterpreted. Maybe one of the treated subjects was experiencing an undetected separate problem and so responded poorly to treatment, while an untreated subject experienced a resurgence of vigor from having just defeated a separate problem, say, a virus or muscle strain.

Maybe feed or water was different enough to bring about an effect. Maybe a medication batch was off.

Nonspecific effects are another driver of apparent improvement. This means that the patient may improve due to aspects around the treatment that are not medically part of the treatment, such as the calm, kind practitioner in a peaceful setting who applies any therapy. The animal's behavior or status may improve, for example, due to the nonspecific effects attendant in the administration of a supplement, touch therapy, or mystical treatment, not from the therapy itself.

If the event occurred outside of a controlled testing situation, that is, if an herb was administered to one ill animal and the animal improved, the logical fallacy of *after the fact, therefore because of the fact* might be misused to identify the herb as the reason for the improvement. The truth is, we don't always know why a sick animal gets better, and we probably don't fully understand the placebo effect either. It has also been suggested that there is no such thing as the placebo response. (Thus complete studies would require three groups: patients receiving the test substance, patients receiving a placebo, and patients receiving nothing.) Other studies expect a placebo effect to improve more than a third of the patients treated.

It is recognized that many patients will improve on their own, that many illnesses tend to come and go, and that good old-fashioned attention—nursing care—will improve many patients. If alternative treatments offered nothing more than special access to the placebo effect, could they be worth trying in many situations?

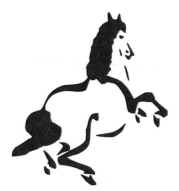

The Smart Consumer

SO HOW DO smart consumers get the best care available for their animals?

Who and what are these chiropractors, naturopaths, homeopaths, and holistic vets? Are they all conventional veterinarians as well? (No.) Do they all practice all of these therapies? (Again, no.)

It is improbable that one could locate any practitioners who offered all alternative treatments, but it is not hard to find a practitioner who decries some or all alternative methods. Often, their reasons for scoffing are more illuminating about the complaining therapist than they are about the touted treatment. Veterinarians who decry all alternatives in favor of strict conventional medicine risk coming off as guarding their empire. On the other hand, when we hear from someone that a remedy works but is not accepted by science because of a power struggle between the established old guard and the new healers, we have to be highly skeptical of the claim. There is no secret conspiracy by modern medicine to block the wide use of wonderful, effective alternative treatments.

Are there red flags that should warn us away from an alternative treatment or practitioner? Yes. Think very carefully about treatments that rely entirely on anecdotes or testimonials for support, and be wary of any medicine or preparation with undisclosed, proprietary, or secret ingredients. Stay skeptical of those who make highly alarmist claims about the malady to be treated or use extraordinary praise, such as "miracle cure," when discussing a treatment. Every therapy or therapist should have a track record with conventional medicine, so be cautious of anyone or anything on which there is very little information available. Practitioners who are hostile to established medicine or reluctant to disclose their education and experience should be looked at with suspicion, as should any who hawk their treatment as the very best available, who suggest delaying necessary veterinary care for your animal, or who claim to cure what modern medicine cannot help at all.

Healthy cynicism requires we reject nearly any treatment that is claimed to always work, yet open-mindedness and sheer reality demand we acknowledge that no one has all the answers. Let's recognize the body as its own healer in most circumstances. Let's recognize the value of the placebo effect without sneering at it. And let us remain wary of both absolute cynicism and absolute belief. Remember, some people have found appreciable success with alternative methods. That alone makes them worth a second look.

AND THE GUINEA PIG

Some holistic practitioners believe inactivity may create hip dysplasia. All good practitioners consider an animal's diet, exercise, and mental health (both stress in his living situation and positive mental stimulation) for causative factors in an ailment. I had a very active, sometimes-lame, four-year-old German shepherd whose veterinarian diagnosed him via radiographs as having hip dysplasia. If I gave a false history of inactivity to alternative practitioners, would they simply suggest I exercise him?

He covered dozens of miles in a week accompanying me on daily hikes, trail runs, or backcountry horse rides; and I played Frisbee with him several times a day. If I could get away with saying he was a couch potato, I would go further. I'd report that he's home alone while I work eighty hours a week and that I feed him the cheapest dog food from the grocery store. Actually, he's rarely alone and is given a high-quality diet. Because I use atypical obedience commands, the dog is unresponsive to strangers trying to command him. He would appear untrained to a vet or other practitioner. I could claim that I just don't have the time or interest to train him. In truth, he's titled at obedience and tracking and has further training in agility, herding, and protection.

Oh, and this dog hates going to the vet. Hates it. Shakes and cries. A veterinarian who advertises his practice as integrating Chinese and contemporary medicine looked at my quivering, whining dog and told me there were earth dogs and water dogs, and one kind just doesn't like the environment of a veterinarian's office. I'm still not clear on whether that vet thinks it's earth dogs or water dogs that don't like going to the vet, but I still think my dog hates clinic settings because he came from death row and it made a negative impression on him. He was pulled from a kill shelter late in the afternoon of his assigned euthanasia day.

On page 339 of veterinarian Cheryl Schwartz's book *Four Paws, Five Directions: A Guide to Chinese Medicine for Cats and Dogs*, she notes dogs with hip dysplasia may be deficient in "kidney jing." Page 35 defines *jing* as "the substantive [sic] essence we are born with." Earlier in her book, Schwartz recounts the theory of five elements as well as the yin and yang organs associated with each element. The author creates a matrix incorporating the time of day an organ works best; the season it's most vulnerable; and the emotions, colors, senses, and body parts to which an organ is related. Sounds, climate, food, odors, and secretions are all half-jokingly factored into an example case: "A dog with itchy red eyes, especially in the spring time, who barks loudly and lunges at the mailman angrily, who craves your chicken dinner and bowl of pasta or your sour ball candy, who has a rancid skin odor, who wakes up every night to scratch at 1:00 AM, and who wants to wear your green T-shirts, you may have a dog with a potential liver problem" (pp. 6–7).

Some of the alternative treatments are on the mystical fringe. What else would alternative practitioners say and recommend for my dog? Would they say he's bored and depressed and his emotional bad health has caused his pain? What variety of treatments would they suggest? More on this later.

A Nonbeliever Goes into the Mystic: Jek and the Psychic

Many nontraditional treatments are difficult to challenge and prove because they are mystical in nature. Supplemental therapies and many touch therapies can be studied, but the mystical offerings are more nebulous. In an effort to be fair, I wanted to explore all options.

Blame it on my mother. She called and said there was an animal psychic in town who was giving readings, and the requested "donation" money was going to a local animal charity.

"You've said you wonder about his past," she reminded me. "Go. It's fun and for a good cause."

Soon Jek was heeling to the back of a pet store where I learned that it wasn't even necessary for me to bring my dog to the reading. This psychic told me she can do readings without the dog present. She can do them by phone or email too.

How about that? I thought. Then she said that Jek, my German shepherd, had no complaints.

"No, I wouldn't expect so," I said, paying my twenty dollars anyway. I wasn't going to let her out of ripping me off. "I'm curious about his past. He came from the pound when he was about a year old."

"He doesn't want to talk about it."

Well, that worked well for the psychic, didn't it? When I said nothing, she went on.

"I think there was a lot of fighting and yelling, and they didn't have time for him. I think he just left, but I'm not sure." She told me he knew what I had done for him, taking him in, and that he appreciated it. I thought that wasn't much of a limb she was going out on.

Then she said, "He doesn't understand why you go so long sometimes." She looked at Jek again and turned back to me. "Hours and hours? Is that right? Running?"

Here's the thing: I don't look like a runner, I just don't. And I certainly wasn't dressed like a runner that day. But I had recently been doing four-hour-long runs because I was entered in a 50K. And because I run backcountry trails, I always bring Jek. Bears and cougars and scary rednecks, oh my, are on those trails, and they are no small part of why we adopted Jek when we did.

The psychic was still waiting for me to confirm what she got from the dog, what she didn't understand.

"Yes, we run hours and hours," I admitted.

"Why?"

"It's for a race I'm going to in a few weeks. After that, we'll back down to one- or two-hour runs. Tell him."

"He heard. Does he have to do the race?"

"No. Just me. He won't be coming."

"He says it was raining the last time you two ran for a long time, and he just wanted to go inside. You have, like, a carpet. By a fire? Do you have a fireplace?"

"Yes."

Plenty of homes have fireplaces in this area. It wasn't much of a guess for any so-called psychic.

I didn't say that it had indeed rained for the final two hours of our most recent long run.

"He's a little vain," she told me.

"Is he?"

"He says he's a lot better-looking than your other dog. He says it's not even a contest. What kind is the other dog?"

"A Golden," I answered. Golden retrievers are generally beautiful, but honestly, the one who had moved in with us was obviously badly bred and not a very good example of the breed. We didn't love her for her looks but for her heart, for her personality. Jek, on the other hand, is more along the lines of drop-dead gorgeous. And to hear the psychic tell it, he knows it.

There was more. I wondered how Jek liked his many dog friends, what he thought about our horses, and even what they thought about him. The psychic told me that one of the horses (the one we think is our responsible guy) said Jek was a lot smarter than our other dog (hideously true) but that he didn't understand Jek's ears at first.

I puzzled over that latter comment as I left. A lot of dogs have come to our barn. There are Labs and a beagle, poodles, a Kom, a Rottweiler, floppy-eared mutts, and a pointer. Jek is the only pinnate-eared dog among them. The horse hadn't seen another dog—at least not at our barn—with erect, pointy ears.

And of course, I thought about why. Why, oh why did the psychic venture to say something as far out of the mainstream of good guessing as "Jek doesn't understand why we run for hours and hours?" Although I resist the idea that psychic power enabled her to know something so odd and specific, I cannot explain why she came up with this. I just can't. So would I ever consider trying a psychic for a real problem with an animal? Well, yes.

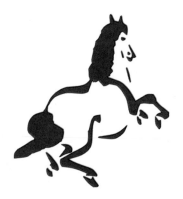

PART 2

THE ALTERNATIVE THERAPIES

Touch, Supplementation, Mystical, and More

EXAMINING THE LIST of alternative treatments practitioners use, we find many similarities and overlapping methods. There are also synonymous terms (such as *zone therapy* and *reflexology*) and differing understandings of the same term. (For example, some reflexologists define the practice as assessment and treatment strictly through the foot, while others expand the theory to the ear.)

Comparison of the alternative treatments is easier when similar treatments are first grouped together. Many of these alternative treatments can obviously be grouped into either noninvasive touch or supplementation. Others fall into a group that can be categorized as mystical, and still others cannot be classified into one of these three preceding categories. People might argue about which category a treatment belongs to, and some therapies fall into more than one category, but all alternative treatments from the alphabetical list presented in the introduction of this book are in at least one of the following four categories: *touch, supplementation, mystical,* and *other* treatments.

And what about the qualifier that some treatments deserve to be in more than one classification? Some of the alternative treatments really can be categorized into more than one of our four groups of treatments. Traditional Chinese veterinary medicine, for example, has aspects of touch, supplementation, mystical, and more. Reiki has both touch and mystical components too.

While the grouping of alternative treatments might not be something all would agree upon, remember this categorization is meant to make understanding therapies with similar components a bit easier,

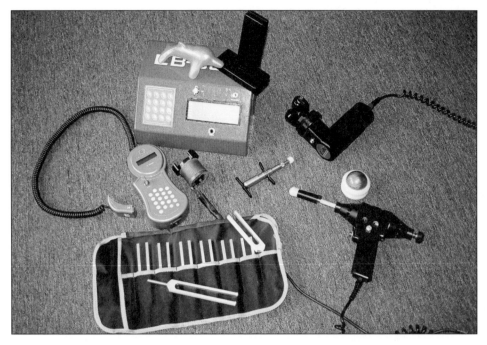

ABOVE: Many different devices have been developed for alternative treatments. Clockwise from bottom left: tuning fork set; cold laser; detoxification unit (magnets on top of detox unit); percussor, manual pressure implement; electric adjustor. Center: manual adjustor.

so that they can be compared and consumers can make informed choices.

Dozens upon dozens of alternative treatments are available for literally every medical and behavioral condition that an animal could suffer.

Acupressure *Touch*

Acupuncture *Other* (see *Special Report: Acupuncture*)

Alpha-Stim *Other* (See MENS Listing)

Anma *Touch*

Apitherapy *Supplementation*

Aquapuncture *Other* (See Acupuncture Listing)

Aquatic Massage Therapy (AMT) *Touch* (See Shiatsu Listing)

Aromatherapy *Other*

Astrology *Mystical*

Augmentation Therapy *Supplementation*

Aura Adjustment *Mystical*

Aural Photography *Other*

Auriculotherapy *Touch* (See Reflexology Listing)

Ayurveda *Other*

Bach Flower Remedies *Supplementation*

Biochemic Tissue Salts *Supplementation* (See Tissue Salts Listing)

Bioplasma *Supplementation* (See Tissue Salts Listing)

Botanicals *Supplementation*

Bowen Technique *Touch*

Cannabis Products *Supplementation*

Cell Salts *Supplementation* (See Tissue Salts Listing)

Cell Therapy *Supplementation* (See Glandular Therapy Listing)

Chakra Adjustment *Mystical*

Chelation Therapy *Supplementation*

Chi/Ji/Ki/Qi Adjustment *Mystical*

Chiropractic *Touch*

Chromotherapy *Other* (See Color Therapy Listing)

Cold Laser *Other* (See Laser Therapy Listing)

Colloidal Minerals *Supplementation*

Colloidal Silver *Supplementation*

Color Therapy *Other*

Craniosacral Therapy *Touch*

Crystal Healing *Mystical*

Cupping *Other*

Dark Field Microscopy (DFM) *Other*

Diatomaceous Earth *Supplementation*

Deep Connective Tissue Massage *Touch* (See Massage Listing)

Deep Muscle Therapy *Touch* (See Massage Listing)

Detoxification Therapy *Other*

Dowsing *Mystical*

Effleurage *Touch*

Electroacupuncture *Other* (See Acupuncture Listing)

Electrodermal Testing *Other*

Electromagnetic Therapy *Other* (See Magnet Therapy Listing)

Electrophoresis *Other*

Endotapping *Touch*

Energy Emission Analysis (EEA) *Other* (See Kirlian Assessment Listing)

Essential Oils *Supplementation*

Extracorporeal Shock Wave Therapy (ESWT) *Other* (See Ultrasonography Listing)

Fascial Manipulation *Touch*

Feng Shui *Mystical*

Flower Essences *Supplementation*

Functional Medicine *Other*

Galvanic Skin Response Scanning *Other* (See Electrodermal Testing)

Gemmotherapy *Supplementation*

Glandular Therapy *Supplementation*

Gold Beads *Other* (See Acupuncture Listing)

Hair Analysis *Other*

Hair Mineral Analysis (HMA) *Other*

Harmonic Medicine (See Tuning Fork Therapy Listing)

Heliotherapy *Other*

Hemp Oil *Supplementation* (See Cannabis Products Listing)

Herbalism *Supplementation*

Homeopathy *Supplementation*

Homotoxicology *Supplementation*

Hydrotherapy *Other*

Hyperbaric Oxygen Treatment (HBOT) *Other*

Hypnosis *Mystical*

Immuno-Augmentive Therapy *Supplementation*

Infrasound *Other*

Infratonic Therapy *Other*

Integrative Manual Therapy (IMT) *Touch*

Intrinsic Data Field Analysis *Other*

Iontophoresis *Other* (See Electrophoresis Listing)

Iridology *Other*

Kinergetics *Other* (See Kinesiology Listing)

Kinesiology *Other*

Kirlian Assessment *Other*

Larval Therapy *Other*

Laser Therapy *Other*

Limbic Massage *Touch* (see T Touch Listing)

Live Blood Analysis *Other* (See Dark Field Microscopy Listing)

Live Cell Therapy *Supplementation* (See Glandular Therapy Listing)

Lomilomi *Touch*

Low Energy Photon Therapy (LEPT) *Other* (See Photonic Therapy Listing)

Low-Level Laser Therapy (LLLT) *Other* (See Laser Therapy Listing)

Maggot Therapy *Other* (See Larval Therapy Listing)

Magnetic Therapy *Other*

Manual Lymph Drain (MLD) *Touch*

Massage *Touch*

Medicinal Mushrooms *Supplementation* (See Botanicals Listing)

Megavitamin Therapy *Supplementation*

Mesenchymal Stromal Cells *Other* (See Stem Cell Listing)

Mesotherapy *Other*

Microcurrent/Microamperage Electrical Neuromuscular Stimulation (MENS) *Other*

Moxibustion *Other*

Muscle Response Testing *Other*

Myofascial Release *Touch*

Nambudripad's Allergy Elimination Technique (NAET) *Other*

Naturopathy *Other*

Neural Therapy *Other*

Neuromuscular Electrical Stimulation (NMES) *Other* (See TENS)

Newcastle Treatment *Other*

Nosodes *Supplementation*

Nutraceuticals *Supplementation*

Nutrigenomics *Other*

Nutrition Therapy *Supplementation*

Orthomolecular Medicine *Supplementation*

Osteopathy *Touch*

Ozone Therapy *Other*

Pendulum Assessment *Mystical* (See Dowsing Listing)

Petrissage *Touch*

Pheromone Therapy *Supplementation*

Photonic Therapy *Other*

Platelet-Rich Plasma *Other* (See Stem Cell Listing)

Polyfrequency Spectrum Testing *Other* (See Reba Testing)

Polysan *Other* (See Sanum Remedies)

Pressure Garments *Other*

Prolotherapy *Other*

Psychosomatic Energetics *Other* (See ReBa Testing)

Psychic Analysis/Communication *Mystical*

Pulsed/Pulsating Electromagnetic Field Therapy (PEMF) *Other*
    (See Magnetic Therapy Listing)

Qigong *Mystical*

Qxci Quantum Healing *Other*

Radionics *Other*

RainDrop Technique *Other*

ReBa Testing *Other*

Reflexology *Touch*

Regenerative Medicine *Other* (See Stem Cell Listing)

Reiki *Mystical*

Rolfing *Touch*

Saliva Testing *Other*

Sanum Remedies *Other*

Scenar *Other*

Sclerotherapy *Other*

Segmental Therapy *Other* (See Neural Therapy Listing)

Shiatsu *Touch*

Sonic Therapy *Other*

Sonography *Other*

Stem Cells *Other*

T'ai Ji *Mystical* (See Qigong Listing)

Therapeutic Touch *Mystical*

Thought Field Therapy (TFT) *Mystical*

Ting Point Therapy *Touch* (See Acupuncture Listing)

Tissue Salts *Supplementation*

Tongue-Pulse Diagnosis *Other*

Traditional Chinese Medicine/Traditional Chinese Veterinary Medicine (TCM/TCVM) *Other*

Transcutaneous Electrical Neuromuscular Stimulation (TENS) *Other*

Trigger Point Therapy *Touch*

Ttouch *Touch*

Tui Na *Touch*

Tuning Fork Therapy *Touch*

Ultrasonography *Other*

Urotherapy *Supplementation*

Veterinary Orthopedic Manipulation (VOM) *Touch*

Vibrational Therapy *Mystical*

Vita Flex *Mystical*

Water (Acidified, Activated, Alkalinized, Clustered, Energized, Hexagonal, Inducted, Ionized, Live, Oxygenated, Pentagonal, Structured) *Supplementation*

Watsu *Touch* (See Shiatsu Listing)

Zero Balancing *Mystical*

Most alternatives on the above list are treatments, but some are diagnostic. While the diagnostic methods are not therapeutic, they are still alternative in nature because they are not methods accepted by the general community of conventional medicine.

Let's examine these alternatives and their multiple permutations from the view of both skeptic and believer, with an attempt to find common ground. Accepting what cannot be explained can go hand in hand with debunking when the primary goal is simply to gain knowledge.

Special Report: Acupuncture

LET'S BEGIN AT the beginning of our original alphabetical list: acupressure and acupuncture. Acupressure is acupuncture done with manual pressure instead of needles. Acupuncture is such a cornerstone of alternative care that it deserves a special look. So what is acupuncture, where does it come from, and what does it do?

Acupuncture advocates point to a Chinese tradition of healing going back thousands of years. The late Robert Imrie DVM, along with Wally Sampson DVM, David Rámey DVM, and Paul Buell PhD (a historian of Chinese medicine) give a different time line on the emergence of acupuncture and traditional Chinese medicine.

They report that the earliest known Chinese veterinary piece, *Qinan Yaoshu*, dating from the sixth century, does not mention acupuncture, while existing works on human medicine do refer to qi. (*Qi* can be defined as an invisible life force believed by practitioners to exist.) The first works mentioning acupuncture date from the

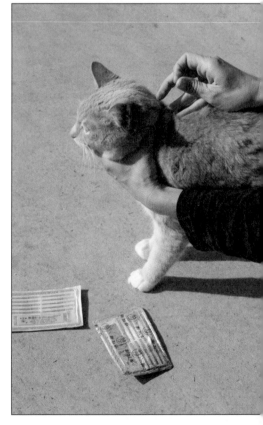

BELOW: **Acupuncture is one of the most well-studied alternative treatments.**

fifth or eighth century, although these may be referencing *Huangdi neijing*, which might date from 200 BC. Needling, meaning to bleed a patient, is first mentioned in the 1608 work *Yuan Heng liaoma ji*, but that text has nothing like the modern understanding of specific meridians targeted by fine needles. (Meridians can be defined as channels along which practitioners believe qi flows.) The idea of bleeding a patient was common to many cultures, including early European medical efforts that predate the modern understanding of physiology. In the 1800s, both China and Japan banned acupuncture as they tried to adopt modern medicine. With the rise of the Maoist government and China's purging of all things foreign, the term *traditional Chinese medicine* was first heard in the west. In the early 1930s, a Chinese doctor named Cheng Dan'an moved acupuncture points away from blood vessels, repositioning the points over nerves, thus moving needling away from bloodletting and into an idea of stimulating nerve points or qi. A Frenchman, Georges Soulié de Morant wrote *Chinese Acupuncture* in 1939, identifying meridians. In 1957 French doctor Paul Nogier invented additional Chinese therapy and termed it traditional medicine.

Imrie, Sampson, et alia, point out that *Veterinary Acupuncture: Ancient Art to Modern Medicine* (Allen Schoen, DVM, editor [Mosby, 1994]) notes that meridians and acupuncture points, now taught as part of traditional Chinese medicine, originated around the 1970s at the insistence of Westerners. They further highlight an admission by authors of another modern text with the same title (Alan M. Klide, DVM, and Shiu H. Kung, PhD, *Veterinary Acupuncture* [University of Pennsylvania Press, 1977]) that there is no information on small animal acupuncture in ancient China. Klide and Kung quote from the 1972 *Chinese Veterinary Handbook* (produced by the Lan Chou Veterinary Research Institute in Gan Shu, China), which does not discuss modern acupuncture, but rather bleeding, cauterizing, and draining with needles.

The recent history reported above flies in the face of the many practitioners who tout traditional Chinese veterinary medicine

(TCVM) and its purported ancient history. Numerous tests have been conducted to try to determine if acupuncture does positively affect patients, and the results have been variable. And yet, in *Love, Miracles, and Animal Healing*, Allen Schoen, DVM, recounts resuscitating a dog—in an emergency room setting after nine conventional veterinarians and technicians gave up on the animal—with acupuncture on a special point (although he does not reveal the location of the point).

One of the strongest criticisms of traditional Chinese medicine is its concept of *qi*, mentioned above, believed to be an intangible life force. Recall the ancient Greek concept of the four humors and their corresponding seasons and personalities. Are the two concepts equally valid folk understandings? Some acupuncturists don't necessarily believe in the notion of qi, but they perform fine needling, saying it sometimes works, but they don't know why.

A method of conducting double-blind studies in acupuncture has been developed. A device with an opaque sheath inserts a needle when a plunger is pressed, and there is a look-alike device that does not insert a needle. In studies, the acupuncturist depresses a plunger but does not know if the plunger is inserting a needle into the skin or if a blunt wood needle merely pushes against the skin. Human patients have proved to be unable to tell whether they have been pricked by a needle or felt the poke from a blunt wood object. Studies have shown no difference in effect between patients that have received the needles-into-the-skin versus patients who only felt the equivalent of pricks from a wooden toothpick. Human patients who feel better after acupuncture treatment may be benefiting from what are termed nonspecific effects—the expectation of benefit, the therapeutic setting, and the session dedicated to the patient's wellness all combine to make the patient feel better.

Acupuncture procedures are recommended more and more often for behavioral disorders, pain management, and many other medical problems. Massachusetts's prestigious Tufts Cummings School of Veterinary Medicine now offers a course in acupuncture even while acupuncture is not accepted by a great deal of the scientific community. Other veterinary schools offer significant coursework and study in CAM too. While Imrie and his colleagues admit that acupuncture studies have a slight positive edge, they say better-controlled studies tend to have negative results.

But must we throw out the baby with the bathwater? Remember the couple whose dog would not let his scraped legs heal until after receiving acupuncture? We cannot ignore the many satisfied patients of acupuncture. We can make an informed choice.

Even if the concept of specific acupoints and meridians is a new invention, the slight positive edge documented in some acupuncture studies remains. The fact that the reason for the edge remains unexplained need not dissuade someone interested in trying the treatment for their animal. Human medicine has documented but failed to thoroughly explain the existence of referred pain—for example, heart attack victims often experience pain down their left arms or up into their jaws. There are things we don't yet understand and things we may never understand. As comprehension grows, treatment generally evolves and acupuncture continues to be recommended by some practitioners for a very wide array of complaints. The American Holistic Veterinary Medical Association notes several different certifications for practitioners. (See this book's resources section.)

Can an acupuncturist who is trained on people work on a horse, dog, or cat without special training to work on animals? It certainly happens, but generally it is better to have a specialist who is trained and practices specifically on animals. Alternative medicine is rife with many created meridian maps and body drawings superimposed over ears, feet, or hands and then transferred between different species. One wonders if an acupuncturist trained to work on people might try to target a horse's gallbladder meridian not knowing that horses have no gallbladder.

Acupuncture remains one option, but our list of alternative treatments needs to be explored. Whether alternative treatments are viewed skeptically or with an open mind, there is an amazing range of options.

Touch Therapies

THE POWER OF touch, the kindness of a caress, has an undeniable positive effect. While the benefits are difficult to measure, on a subjective level, there is no doubt that pleasant massage feels . . . pleasant. Some forms of manual physical therapy can be decidedly uncomfortable, and some have mystical components that may or may not conflict with a client's belief system. Many, although classified as a touch therapy, also could be classified as mystical energy treatments, such as the Bowen technique and kinesiology, or could be classified as a whole medicine system, such as chiropractic or TCVM. Both auriculotherapy and reflexology are touch treatments that are first theoretically diagnostic in nature, thus not wholly a touch therapy.

Ancient and new touch treatments overlap each other at times, leaving a lot of options.

While evidence-based medicine is unable to report hard definitions of improvement in animals who receive touch therapies, scientists would not generally refute the simple line of reasoning that an animal who is cared for and appreciates attention is likely to be less stressed and may have a healthy edge on an animal who does not receive any form of massage or physical therapy. For animals who do seem to enjoy the handling, and clients who have the funds to experiment, there is little reason not to try a treatment that doesn't conflict with their beliefs. Side effects are uncommon in most manual physical therapies, although injuries have been reported in geriatric patients, especially those with degenerative disorders.

ACUPRESSURE

See the above special report on acupuncture. Various practitioners report acupressure points may be stimulated manually, with pressure device or via lasers, lights, or tuning forks.

ANMA

Also transliterated hyphenated (*an-ma*) or as two words (*an ma*), *anma* is the Japanese word for "press and rub." Anma massage is characterized by a kneading manipulation attempting to restore chi. The treatment may be performed on acupressure points and is done dry, without oil or other lubrication.

BOWEN TECHNIQUE

Australian Tom Bowen developed the Bowen technique: intervals of gentle massage by finger and thumb pressure followed by specific rest intervals, usually two minutes in length. Practitioners believe that the rest period allows energy released to travel throughout the body and that the technique benefits numerous physical and mental problems. After the first body area is worked and rested, the practitioner moves to a new area. Before he died in 1982, Tom Bowen adapted his method to animal treatment and trained other practitioners in the technique.

CHIROPRACTIC

Literally meaning "done by hand," classical chiropractic is the manual manipulation of the spinal joints through short, rapid thrusts in an effort to adjust what the practitioner believes are very minor subluxations that are believed by chiropractors to cause disease and all manner of ailments. It is often used for animals who have suffered a fall or other trauma, for example from a traffic accident. Instruments and devices are used by some chiropractors to make adjustments.

See the therapists section, *What Is a Chiropractor?*

CRANIOSACRAL THERAPY

Based on a belief that the fused skull bones are actually movable and the cerebrospinal fluid surrounding the brain and spine are actively pumped and receptive to very light manual pressure by the practitioner, craniosacral therapy is a touch therapy, although it—and

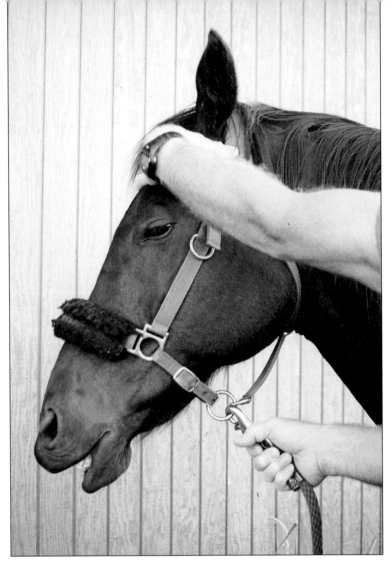

ABOVE: **Craniosacral therapy. Can the skull bones on this reportedly hard-headed horse be moved with manual pressure?**

many touch therapies, including those listed above—could be classified as *other* due to the conflict between its fundamental hypothesis and modern physiological understanding. Practitioners report animals seem to relax and enjoy the treatment.

ENDOTAPPING

Gentle repeated physical tapping, called tapotement, has been used in a number of physical therapies, including in accepted scientific medical applications, such as when a pediatric patient is tapped either by the therapist's cupped hands or with a small percussive device clapping on the patient's chest to loosen lung secretions.

Endotapping, also written endo-Tapping, is a manual therapy applied in an effort to relax an animal and thus enhance a training session. It is applied either during or directly before the training. The technique

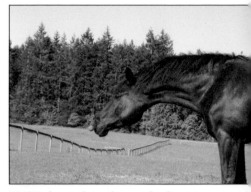

ABOVE: **In endotapping, animals are often initially resistant.**

was conceived by Jean-Philippe Giacomini about twenty-five years ago after he noticed a horse relaxing after he patted it.

While a modified dressage whip or a wand made of wood or synthetic material may be used for endotapping, the device Giacomini developed is called an Endo-stick. The endo-stick, also written endostick, enhances the practitioner's reach, and has a small foam ball on the end that taps the animal. Giacomini believes that animals release endorphins while being tapped with the endostick.

Tapping with an endostick usually begins on the animal's neck or back. Taps are kept in the same area initially but may graduate to taps all over the animal's body. The tapping is done at a slow steady rate, and the animal's emotional response is monitored closely. It is key that the animal begin to relax under the tapping. If the animal avoids or otherwise resists the tapping, the therapist or trainer gently continues until the animal displays the desired acceptance and relaxes while being tapped.

Giacomini points out that horses, being prey animals, must be in a parasympathetic state to truly benefit from a physical rehabilitation or training session. (The parasympathetic nervous system is the counterpart of the sympathetic system; the latter is the body's up-regulator providing an animal's fight-or-flight reactivity, while the parasympathetic is the down-regulator.) Certainly, many horse trainers want to see a horse licking or chewing as an indicator that it has begun to relax or to think about a training session. Stimulation of the parasympathetic nervous system, usually through a primary nerve called the vagus nerve, is associated with salivation, which explains why a horse in a parasympathetic state would lick and work its mouth to accommodate increased salivation.

Detractors of endotapping have termed the tapping to be an annoying sensation, or merely a distraction. In clinics, some therapists have demonstrated good results with overcoming, for example, a horse's recalcitrance to perform a desired feat, or to improve one-sided stiffness.

Predictably, the treatment has been extended across species. A dog with a fear of thunder is one example of an animal who may be treated with endotapping. A similar physical therapy is sometimes simply called tapping or the tap method.

In another example, a horse with scarred legs from a foalhood entanglement in a wire fence was brought to a training session to work on her apparent fear of tight confinement. The mare could be difficult to load into a trailer, and seemed fearful when being asked by a rider to step lightly against a gate to enable the rider to open and close the gate while mounted. The horse was endotapped prior to further training, but the rider reported no obvious difference in outcome between a regular training session versus sessions preceded by endotapping.

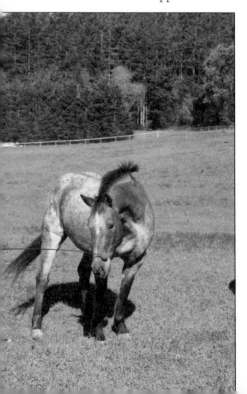

LEFT: **Horse trainers want to see a horse lick or otherwise activate its mouth as an indication that it is thinking, relaxing, or absorbing a session; not all trainers realize that salivation is indicative of parasympathetic stimulation.**

INTEGRATIVE MANUAL THERAPY

Integrative manual therapy (IMT) is a form of physical assessment and massage developed and trademarked by Sharon Weiselfish Giammatteo, PhD, for human patients. IMT has spread to animal practitioners and is often compared to myofascial release and Rolfing, or other forceful touch therapies.

Some IMT practitioners refer to their work as integrative manual therapies when they offer numerous, overlapping services, such as chiropractic, ultrasound, massage, herbs, homeopathy, et cetera.

Doctors usually use the acronym *IMT* when referring to a condition called immune-mediated thrombocytopenia, a specific form of thrombocytopenia (low platelets), so it is important to be clear when using the acronym.

LOMILOMI

A Hawaiian massage technique, lomilomi has also been adapted to animal treatment although there are relatively few practitioners available. Some therapists invoke a mystical component into the treatment while other lomilomi practitioners do not. While early lomilomi givers may well have prayed while massaging, it was common in the old culture to combine praying with most activities, thus modern lomilomi can simply be a deep massage, sometimes performed by more than one practitioner at a time on the same animal patient.

MANUAL LYMPH DRAIN

Manual lymph draining (MLD) is intended to assist the body's lymphatic system in draining. Proponents suggest that the physical stimulation of massage increases lymph flow, thus aiding the body in self-cleansing. While there is no doubt that the massage can be enjoyable and relaxing, it cannot be demonstrated to detoxify the patient through enhanced lymph drainage. MLD may be beneficial, but maybe not for the reasons believed by its adherents.

MASSAGE

The mainstay of touch therapies, general massage has been practiced essentially throughout the world. It is more than petting the animal when done for specific therapeutic intent, and it is an accepted tool to induce trust and bonding. One theory suggests that animals who are massaged frequently when they are young will produce fewer stress hormones as they age, which will in turn help the animal's health.

Massage therapists identify different applications, such as *deep connective tissue massage* or *deep muscle therapy*, to indicate a specialty they provide or a recommendation for an animal. *Effleurage* is a massaging stroke done with the hand flat, initially in slow passes. It is often used in the beginning of a massage session. *Petrissage* is a deeper massage, characterized by kneading and rolling the skin and, indirectly, the muscles. Therapists may also use tools, such as chilled stones (cryotherapy) or heated rocks, towels, or other items to impart a different feel to the massage.

Regulations governing animal massage therapists vary greatly from one region to another. Some American states require therapists to first be certified as human massage therapists with several hundred hours or training, some require therapists to work under a veterinarian's direction, and some are unregulated. Practitioners may skirt legal requirements by promoting their service as bodywork other than massage.

MYOFASCIAL RELEASE

Similar to the idea of fascial manipulation, and taking trigger points a step further, myofascial release is a massage that involves physical stretching and manipulation combined with cross-friction work in an attempt to alleviate adhesions and inelasticity in the tough connective tissue (fascia) around muscles. It can be uncomfortable but is often recommended for animals who have developed excessive stiffness, especially with old injuries. See *Fascial Manipulation* and *Rolfing*.

Myofascial Release, Trigger Points, and Dead Tissue

The older, gaited mare had been lacking in impulsion, reluctant to move forward off the leg, and generally recalcitrant. An equine massage practitioner worked for two hours on the old mare's neck. After just one session, the horse's attitude improved remarkably, and she moved out. She went back to work at her job as a lesson and trail horse for very young children.

The owner was certain the massage had improved the horse. This is a subjective assessment, but one we trust when we trust the general competence of the speaker. If animals could talk with human language, we could ask clearly how they felt before and after the treatment, indeed how it felt while the treatment occurred.

I asked the happy owner exactly what kind of massage the equine massage therapist had administered to the old gaited mare.

"Myofascial release."

I scheduled a myofascial release session, making myself an additional animal case study: homo sapien, the author, a middle-aged recreational runner who limped into a physical therapist's office, legs sparking with pain.

The therapist reefed on my calves.

"Ow! What is that all about?"

"Myofascial release. You need it."

She did cross-friction around my knees. Again, ow.

Next she pushed one fingertip into my thigh. It felt as though she bore in with all her power, though my skin was merely dented around her fingertip. Soon, it felt like she backed off, and I thanked her.

Smiling, she told me she'd kept the same pressure, but that she was touching a trigger point. The point had turned off and that's why I felt relief, as though she'd finally eased her pressure. She touched again and again, switching off hyperreactive muscles.

Later, I received more trigger point therapy from a massage practitioner. I asked how she knew where to touch to find these trigger points.

She grimaced. "It feels like dead tissue."

Like the physical therapist, her fingertips could palpate a difference in the feel of different sections of tissue.

Receiving myofascial release and trigger point therapy was always painful, but after the treatment, my legs felt so much better. They felt quiet, rested, ready to run ten miles.

Massage as a whole is a therapy that straddles the two worlds of alternative treatments and science-based medicine. Practitioners offer an enormous variety of theories, methods, and situations in which they recommend massage therapy.

A top equine veterinarian told me about a horse he examined that he determined needed colic surgery while an alternative practitioner suggested massage instead.

Colic is a lay term for intestinal distress. In severe equine colic, the horse's gut quits working correctly. The horse does not pass digested food. The material can rot, and the intestinal wall can become permeable and leak. Yards and yards of the horse's gut can literally die while still in the body. Surgery removes the necrotic (dead) tissue, saving the horse from lethal infection.

But the owner of the colic horse was swayed by the consult of the alternative practitioner and elected to have the horse's inflamed and impacted gut treated simply with external massage.

The colic horse died.

OSTEOPATHY

Andrew Taylor Still, an American physician who practiced in the late 1800s and early 1900s, is the father of osteopathy. He theorized that the musculoskeletal system could intrinsically overcome ailments and developed the manual touch treatment that would become known as *osteopathic manipulative medicine (OMM)*, or osteopathic manipulative treatment. OMM is similar to chiropractic manipulation but does not focus so exclusively on the spine and other joints.

In human medicine, osteopathy was the medical field that competed essentially on par with advances in modern medicine, to the point that doctors of osteopathy and medical doctors are largely synonymous terms.

Osteopathy and OMM soon came to animal care. Osteopathic care is sporadically available to pets in the United States. In the United Kingdom, osteopaths may belong to the Association of Chartered Physiotherapists in Animal Therapy and require a referral from a veterinarian before treating an animal.

REFLEXOLOGY

Formerly called *zone therapy*, reflexology is the theory that the body can be mapped on the foot, although some proponents extend this effort to the animal's ear (known as *auriculotherapy*, as the outer ear appendage is called the auricle). Specific areas of the foot are thought to correspond to various organs and those areas are believed to be susceptible to manipulation from the corresponding area in the foot. Obviously the preceding could classify reflexology as *other*, not a touch therapy, but it is categorized here due to the massage aspect that is performed in treatment. (Note that *zone therapy* can also refer to a specific early chiropractic spin-off.)

One concern with accepting the idea of one body part being a representative microsystem of the entire body is the disparity in the various available charts attempting to map the body onto the foot or ear (or iris, in the case of iridology). A South African veterinary study of auriculotherapy had mixed results.

Reflexology does have both diagnostic and therapeutic goals. First the foot is examined to assess overall health, as the reflexologists believe various sections of the paw correspond to organs and systems, thus can be assessed through examining the animal's foot. The foot is then massaged to treat the part of the body the practitioner's examination determined is in need of treatment.

Among animal therapists, the usual practice is on a dog's paw. Reflexology is essentially palm reading (followed by touch therapy)

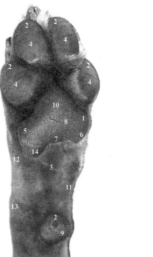

1-bladder
2-brain
3-circulation
4-eye
5-heart
6-hip
7-intestine
8-kidney
9-liver
10-lungs
11-ovaries/testes
12-shoulder
13-spine
14-stomach

ABOVE: **Reflexologists disagree about what areas of the foot might represent which organs and other body systems.**

done on the paw (or ear, with auriculotherapy), with health instead of fortune being the topic.

ROLFING

Biochemist Ida Pauline Rolf, a peer of Moshé Feldenkrais, developed the concept of *structural integration* (later called Rolfing). Rolfing is a treatment based on the idea that the body can be realigned through a myofascial massage that improves motion as well as emotion. Therapists soon adapted Rolfing to horses and dogs, particularly recommending it for sports injuries and other gait or back problems. See *Fascial Manipulation* and *Myofascial Release*.

SHIATSU

The Japanese term for finger-pressure, *shiatsu* is an outgrowth of anma and Japanese acupressure. It focuses more on stress reduction and prevention than on reactive healing. Practitioners use their fingertips and thumbs to apply gentle pressure in an effort to stimulate what they believe is the animal's vital force. Therapists who do not subscribe to the notion of vital force point to the manual manipulation stimulating blood flow and promoting muscle relaxation. Initially more commonly practiced on dogs, there are now shiatsu practitioners for horses as well.

Shiatsu is sometimes done with both patient and therapist immersed in warm water, a combination sometimes called Watsu, or aquatic massage therapy, and is increasingly encountered as indoor canine spas become more common.

TRIGGER POINT THERAPY

Also called *trigger point myotherapy*, trigger point therapy treats hypersensitive areas in a muscle or the fascia surrounding the muscle. These oversensitive areas are thought to develop in response to injuries or strains that could have gone unnoticed, such as a fall, impact, or overextension, for example when a horse slips in mud or a dog roughhouses with a playmate.

Skilled therapists can sometimes locate an active trigger point through palpation alone, though usually the animal gives an indication of pain at the area. Often there is referred pain, that is, the point of pain in a shoulder muscle can indicate joint strain some distance away.

In the 1940s, trigger point injection therapy was done with small injections of saline or lidocaine to the painful point, but physical therapists soon felt they could achieve good results with manual manipulation. In successful treatment, trigger points are essentially turned off and the muscle is restored to a normal state. Because the treatment can be uncomfortable, especially early on, it may not be well tolerated by some animals.

TTOUCH

Canadian Linda Tellington-Jones adapted *Feldenkrais*, a movement and awareness therapy for humans developed by Moshe Feldenkrais, to animals. TTouch can be considered both a training and treatment tool. The aim is to retrain the brain and the body to alleviate what are essentially bad physical habits in the way an animal moves. While originally caused by pain, stress, or fear, poor movement can later become habitual and problematic. Limping is an example of pain that can become habitual, such as someone with an old knee injury who continues to unnecessarily favor one leg while climbing or descending stairs, for example. Animals can develop similar habits of poor motion.

TTouch generally consists of gentle, circular massage in a rhythmic pattern that is performed all over the animal's body in an effort to promote awareness, circulation, and relaxation. Different types of touches are taught for different circumstances and different species of animals. Trainers and zoo animal caretakers have reported benefits from the treatment.

TTouch is referred to by some as a limbic system massage due to its effort to retrain. Used here, limbic refers to the limbic system—brain structures around the hypothalamus concerned with affective sensations such as pleasure and pain.

TTouch is often combined with additional training methods called TEAM, which alternatively stands for Tellington-Jones Every Animal Method or Tellington-Jones Equine Awareness Method. The method has been criticized for its use of physiognomy (assessing character traits from facial features, for example).

Interestingly, hair whorls, a seemingly innocuous physical trait, may come from the same gene that is responsible for an animal's sidedness (with sidedness referring to the being's preferring to use one side, in the same manner that humans are generally right-handed or left-handed). It could be that an assessment of certain physical features beyond conformation (such as whorls) can aid in the understanding, and thus training, of some animals.

TUI NA

An instructor from one of the United States' top TCVM schools characterized tui na as Chinese chiropractic. Sometimes hyphenated as *tui-na*, the manipulation aims to improve the function of tendons, bones, and joints. It is one of the five main branches of TCVM—see the full section on TCVM.

TUNING FORK THERAPY

Some acupressure practitioners employ tuning forks to deliver pressure to treatment points. One animal chiropractor suggested always using the C note tuning fork because it was the "earth frequency." Called Acutonics by one school and its practitioners, tuning fork therapy has been used postoperatively for animals recovering from surgery, but it remains relatively uncommon.

Tuning forks are also used as a modality apart from any form of acupressure, in hopes of healing with the sound generated by the fork. This is sometimes referred to as harmonic medicine. While this

BELOW: **Acupressure points may be stimulated via needles, electricity, lights, lasers, tuning forks (shown here), injections, or manual pressure.**

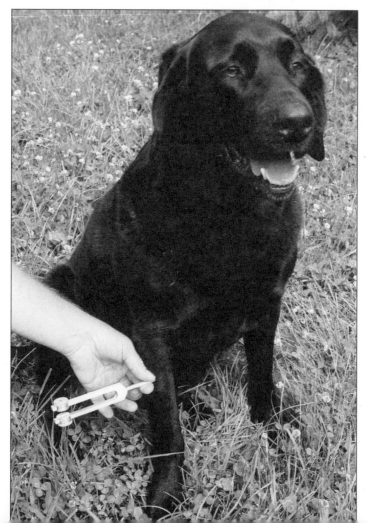

therapy is classified as a touch therapy because it involves touching the patient with the activated tuning forks, it could also be classified as *other* in that the modality attempting to promote healing—sound— is not a touch therapy.

VETERINARY ORTHOPEDIC MANIPULATION (VOM)

Veterinarian William Inman developed VOM, a device-assisted adjusting technique, in 1982. Inman posits neurological interference as a common factor in most disease states, and he uniquely distinguishes between subluxations and luxations to explain this. Conventional medicine defines luxations as dislocations and subluxations as incomplete or partial dislocations. VOM defines a subluxation as a condition of the nervous tissue, not of the bones or joints. Thus, VOM practitioners find subluxations they say are not visible on radiographs, though the luxations' effects are sometimes visible radiographically.

A supporter of chiropractic theory, Inman believes many veterinarians fail to treat anatomical subluxations, and he claims 80 percent of animals have neuronal subluxations. He finds manual chiropractic treatment too slow, especially on uncooperative animals, and he uses a spinal hammer that imparts minute, rapid motion to a very specific treatment area. The stainless steel device, called a spinal accelerometer, is used first diagnostically to read an animal's response, then therapeutically.

Orthopedic problems, such as osteochondritis dissecans (OCD) and canine wobbler syndrome (instability in the skull-cervix joint, or intra-cervical joints) resulting in balance problems and other neurological deficits) as well as conditions not generally regarded as having an orthopedic etiology, such as gastric dilatation-torsion (bloat), are all treated with VOM.

The American Holistic Veterinary Medical Association recognizes VOM as a specialty certification. There are several thousand VOM practitioners to be found in the United States, Canada, Australia, New Zealand, the U.K., and beyond.

Supplementation Therapies

SUPPLEMENTATION IS A very broad field. The primary factor placing an alternative treatment in this category is that the treatment being examined is a substance prepared in hope of benefiting the animal's well-being and administered (topically, orally, or via another route) as a health supplement.

Many herb preparations, especially Chinese herbs, are actually formulas, that is, not a preparation made from just one herb but from several different, often undisclosed, origins.

Other supplements might equally be classified as mystical treatments, in that the therapy depends upon a belief that there is something of value other than plain water in the preparation, but they are classed here as supplements because they meet the bare criteria of being a substance administered, usually topically or orally, in hope of benefiting the animal's health.

BELOW: Varieties of the potentially dangerous hawthorn (*Crataegus*) have long been used in the folk medicine of Europe and the Americas for the heart and blood, and in China for the digestive system.

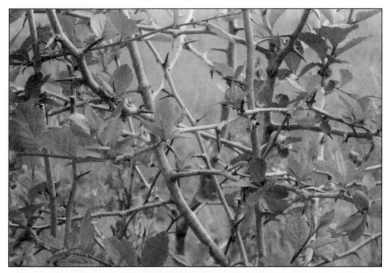

There are significant regulatory battles within the supplement industry that affect consumers. *The New York Times* reported in May 2010 that an investigation by the U.S. Congress found many herbal supplements to be contaminated with heavy metals or pesticides. In response, a trade organization that represents the supplement industry, the Council for Responsible Nutrition, pointed out that trace amounts of metals are naturally found in soils. In September 2010, *Consumer Reports* published a warning on twelve supplements (aconite, bitter orange, chaparral, colloidal silver, coltsfoot, comfrey, country mallow, geranium, greater celandine, kava, lobelia, and yohimbe) to be avoided because risks outweighed possible benefits.

Animals' dietary requirements vary not just between the species (the carnivorous cat has extremely different needs than does the herbivorous horse) but according to the animal's individual needs based upon its age and work. One should never simply interchange supplements between animals without professional advice.

Science's difficulty in assessing many of these supplemental treatments is that there are so many compounds in a given supplement. A plant, for example, has very numerous identified and possibly unidentified compounds, and these factors are variable depending upon the plant part (root, stem, leaf, flower), soil condition, season, and processing of the plant. Also, one animal can process various supplements differently than another due to different body chemistry at the time of supplementation as well as other health factors.

Consider vitamins and minerals, for example. Iron absorption is aided by vitamin C, but excess vitamin C hampers the body's absorption of copper. Excess vitamin B1 can lead to deficiency in B2 and B6. Too little vitamin E impairs absorption of selenium, while too much selenium is easily toxic. A plant grown in one area can be toxic with selenium while the same plant grown in different soils might be deficient in this trace mineral. Horse owners work to balance the calcium:phosphorus ratio in the hay, as alfalfa has high calcium and other grasses tend to have much less.

Like other alternatives, supplements may be seen as ranging from mere hype to the truly helpful. Take care to not experiment on your animal, and consider the pros and cons of a treatment with conventional guidance in mind. Gastric distress, allergic reactions, and toxicosis are the most common side effects in supplementation. While supplementation is usually oral, it can also be applied topically, with some products, such as colloidal silver, being applied either orally or topically. Remember that even topically applied alternative supplements can have unintended negative consequences. For example, cats and dogs have been poisoned by the use of pennyroyal oil as a flea and tick deterrent.

Topical Application: The Cyborg Horse

The little black Thoroughbred did well enough, finishing first in enough purses to let his owners be regularly photographed in the winner's circle; placing and showing (coming in second and third, respectively) enough to keep the promise of money alive.

He was smaller than most of his competitors, fifteen hands and two inches, but his owner said, "He had more heart than any other racehorse I ever had."

And more spirit. The little beast—amped up on the hard training, high-grain diet and stall life of a racehorse—once broke loose in the saddling area at the track, sending people running for safety as he careened about, a one-horse circus, every buck punctuated with a staccato release of gas.

The growth arrived suddenly, a nasty, lumpy mass burbling from his eyelid and surrounding skin until it overtook his right eye.

No one knew what had caused the mass, and no one could make it stop. If it was viral, no one wanted their horses around the little guy.

Soon the hideous growth looked artificial, as though a Hollywood makeup artist had created an unnatural horse-plus-something-else from another planet.

"He looked like a cyborg," one veterinarian recalled. "A 'borg horse."

The cyborg gelding was scheduled to be put down. A one-eyed horse can be unsafe on the track, and a gelding has no breeding value. Still shy of his fifth birthday, the 'borg gelding wasn't even at full maturity, but he was suddenly living his last days. Had he been healthy, his post-racing fate would have been retirement to a new career, such as dressage or jumping, but cyborg horses are hard to adopt out, and even harder to sell.

Euthanasia was the answer for the horse with the most heart.

Then his owner tried one more veterinarian, a woman who embraced alternative treatments. This vet regularly recommended homeopathic preparations to her clients, offered chiropractic on many animals, and worked with acupuncturists.

"She had some special salve she said she could put on it," the owner reported. "I told her to go ahead. Nothing else had worked."

The vet topically applied the product, treating the growth repeatedly with a salve no one else had.

And then?

"The growth went away, disappeared completely," the owner told me. "The horse was fine. She saved him." And saved him quickly. Her course of treatment didn't take long, and soon the healthy retired racehorse was off to a rehabilitation and adoption facility.

I asked the alternative veterinarian what was in the salve she put on the little black gelding.

"It was a combination of things," she said mysteriously.

When I pressed further, it turned out she didn't know all of the ingredients in the potion.

I wanted to buy a bottle of the magic salve, read the label, contact the manufacturer. However, the vet told me she could no longer get the product.

Readers are cautioned to seek competent veterinary care for skin lesions on horses. Pyogranuloma (proud flesh) can look quite similar to a fibroblastic sarcoid, but the two have opposite management strategies, and each condition will be worsened by the wrong management. See the University of Liverpool's excellent brief by Dr. Derek Knottenbelt (http://www.liv.ac.uk/sarcoids).

But the little black Thoroughbred no longer looked like a cyborg. His vision was restored, and he enjoyed a long life as a saddle horse.

APITHERAPY

Apitherapy, the administration of honeybee products for health, has an ancient and varied history. Conventional medicine uses insect venom in careful, restricted application for treatment of hypersensitivity. In the realm of alternative treatments, honey, pollen, propolis, royal jelly, and venom have all been used in hope of improved joint function and nutrition, as well as decreased pain and degeneration. Respiratory, integumentary, and dental problems have all been treated with apitherapy; and all have some anecdotal support while generally lacking strong support from scientific research. An exception to this is the fact that honey is bacteriostatic, meaning that microorganisms such as bacteria cannot reproduce in it.

Honey is used topically on wounds as well as ingested. Honey believed to be collected from numerous types of plants is called a multifloral honey, while a honey believed to be collected from only one type of flower is called a monofloral honey. Manuka, collected from the manuka myrtle, which is also called the New Zealand tea tree or leptospermum scoparium, is an example of a

BELOW: **Honey has bacteriostatic properties.**

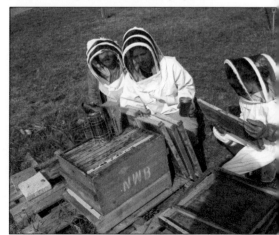

monofloral honey. Advocates believe raw honey contains additional beneficial trace substances. It is certain that honey can be a beneficial topical on a wound; however unprocessed (raw) honey contains many impurities such as bug fragments. A mix of sugar and iodine is a common home hoof infection preparation as the sugar environment does provide some protection for topical infections, but it is not clear that honey-dine (honey and iodine) or sugar and iodine are is more effective than a commercial antiseptic preparation.

Pollen, gathered by bees as they collect nectar from flowers, is suggested by apitherapy proponents as a nutritional supplement as it does contain carbohydrate (in the form of sugar), fat, protein, and many vitamins and minerals. Pollen also contains insect excrement, fungi, and bacteria. Adverse reactions are not uncommon. One study of human athletes did show a benefit with bee pollen supplementation, in that the supplemented group took fewer sick days.

Propolis, the waxy plant material collected by bees to chock their hives, is sometimes suggested for germ-fighting as a topical preparation or an oral ingestion, often in a gelatin capsule. An antimicrobial effect is reported in a laboratory setting but propolis also supports bacterial growth. Again, any animal sensitive to the plant the propolis was gathered from may have a reaction to the propolis.

Royal jelly is especially subject to misinformation, often advertised in literature advocating apitherapy with the comment that royal jelly is consumed only by the queen bee, when in fact all young bee larvae receive royal jelly. Still the queen bee was fed only royal jelly when she was a larva, and her life span and fertility lead to the alternative treatment of administering royal jelly for all manner of weakness.

Bee venom is suggested as a treatment for inflammation, autoimmune arthritis, and degenerative arthritis. Therapists may have processed venom that is administered with a needle or may position a bee over the body, using a container that exposes the animal to the bee until the animal is stung.

Because allergic reactions are fairly common, due care must be exercised by anyone considering any form of apitherapy.

There is also a homeopathic remedy called apis, or *apis mellifica*, that is crafted from the body of a bee as the original mother tincture. See the therapists section, *What Is a Homeopath?*.

AUGMENTATION THERAPY

Not to be confused with *immuno-augmentive therapy* (or *IAT*, an alternative cancer treatment), *augmentation therapy* is sometimes used interchangeably with the terms *mega-nutrients* and *orthomolecular medicine* as a term for vitamin, mineral, and other nutrient supplementation in an effort to help an animal. Preventing, correcting, and reversing pathology is the goal.

BACH FLOWER REMEDIES

Edward Bach, an English medical doctor, turned from science to intuition in the 1930s and decided that disease was largely caused by mental states. He developed what he termed flower essences to alleviate problematic mental states he identified after personally suffering these feelings or habits. His essences are not the contemporary understanding of the term *essence* as a highly concentrated tincture or oil, but rather as a preparation made by collecting dew on a flower. Failing that primary method of collection, it is made by placing a cut flower in water and leaving it in the sunlight, or in the absence of sufficient sun, by steeping the flower. The exposed water is then diluted and administered orally or topically to a patient with a specific mental complaint. The remedies are usually packaged in a manner that protects them from additional light exposure. The thirty-eight original Bach flower remedies and their indications for use are as follows.

BACH FLOWER REMEDIES	
Dew Found On:	Intended to Treat:
Agrimony	concealed worry
Aspen	unexplained anxiety
Beech	intolerance
Centaury	submissiveness
Cerato	lack of self-confidence
Cherry Plum	desperation
Chestnut Bud	repeating mistakes
Chicory	being demanding
Clematis	indifference
Crab Apple	shame
Elm	overwhelmed or inadequate
Gentian	discouragement
Gorse	hopelessness
Heather	self-centeredness
Holly	hatred and jealousy
Honeysuckle	nostalgia
Hornbeam	fatigue
Impatiens	impatience
Larch	despondency
Mimulus	anxiety of an identified cause
Mustard	deep depression
Oak	obstinance
Olive	exhaustion
Pine	guilt
Red Chestnut	anticipating trouble
Rock Rose	hysteria
Rock Water	self-denial
Scleranthus	indecision
Star-of-Bethlehem	grief

Sweet Chestnut	anguish
Vervain	fanaticism
Vine	arrogance
Walnut	transition difficulty
Water violet	aloofness
White Chestnut	preoccupation
Wild Oat	dissatisfaction due to lack of direction
Wild Rose	resignation
Willow	resentment

In addition, Bach created a thirty-ninth remedy, called Rescue Remedy, that was a combination of five flower "essences" (cherry plum, clematis, impatiens, rock rose, and Star-of-Bethlehem), which he suggested for trauma and stress conditions. A cream preparation of Rescue Remedy is also available. Some practitioners consider Bach remedies to be a *vibrational therapy* in that they believe the water takes on the flowers' vibrational energy for healing purposes.

In the early 1990s, the University of California Davis School of Veterinary Medicine abandoned its study of Bach flower remedies as the initial results were disappointing.

BELOW: **Dilute dew. Like all homeopathic preparations, Bach flower remedies are diluted beyond a detectable presence of the original preparation.**

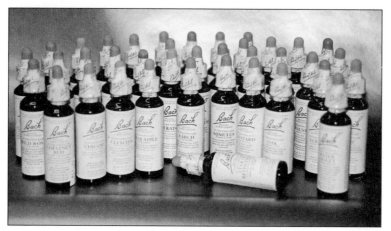

BOTANICAL MEDICINE/ HERBOLOGY

Also called *phytomedicine*, or *herbalism*, this is a vast and ancient field used to treat an extraordinary array of mental and physical complaints. It is not without significant risks, as these organic preparations must be given with care and knowledge. Blue algae, for example, is sometimes recommended as a dietary supplement (spirulina), yet as *microcystic aeruginosa*, it can cause fatal liver damage.

The Physician's Desk Reference for Herbal Medicines, first released in 1998, is a measure of mainstream medicine's recognition of the potential value of many herbal therapies.

The U.S. Food and Drug Administration releases a list of Generally Recognized as Safe items. Hundreds of commonly used herbs are not on this list; for example, two kinds of basil are listed, neither of which is the "holy" basil used in ayurvedic medicine. To add to the confusion, there are very numerous names for many botanicals, with occasional disagreement about which name is attributed to which plant. Thus two practitioners might claim to be giving the same herb but are actually administering different plants, or in the reverse, they could believe they are giving different treatments while they are actually prescribing the same substance. Also, some treatments are known by a common name for an herbal blend.

There are also numerous offshoots of botanical medicine. The American Holistic Veterinary Medical Association distinguishes between specialists in *Western herbs* (*WH*) and *TCVM* herbal practitioners. Some aspects of TCVM are certainly herbalism. The *Red Book of Hergest* is a medieval Welsh text that contains (among much prose and poetry) herbal remedies of the time, and it is sometimes invoked in support of specific herbal remedies suggested.

Gemmotherapy is flower and plant therapy in which only the new buds, shoots, and roots are used, as practitioners believe the newest growth to be the most potent.

Medicinal mushrooms are a relatively understudied treatment, although some reports include immune system—stimulating and cancer-fighting properties, such as Russian Chaga tea. Other fungi are considered antiviral. Polypore mushrooms have significant a history of use in Chinese medicine.

Essiac, a combination of burdock, Indian rhubarb, slippery elm, and sorrel, is an example of a common name for an herbal blend. A Canadian nurse named Renée Caisse began promoting the blend (*essiac* is the reverse spelling of *Caisse*) as a cure for cancer in the 1920s. After her death in 1978, numerous manufacturers began releasing products called essiac. A 1982 study by the Canadian government found no benefit to cancer patients who received essiac.

It is emphasized that herbalism is not a field for hobbyists, as dangers abound. Some plants found in alternative treatment guidebooks (lantana, for example) are also featured in warnings to horse owners about toxic plants. Plants that are safe for one species can be harmful to another. Members of the allium family (chives, onion, garlic, et cetera), so tasty to humans, are toxic to dogs, and especially cats. Alliums contain a disulfide alkaloid that damages their red blood cells and can result in hemolytic anemia.

CANNABIS PRODUCTS (CANNABINIDIOL, CANNABIS OIL, CBD, CBG, CBN, HEMP OIL, ET CETERA)

Cannabis is a robust herb of the *Cannabaceae* family that originated in Asia. Plants of the family include *cannabis sativa*, *cannabis indica*, and *cannabis ruderalis*, with *c. sativa* being the most widely available.

Commonly called marijuana, cannabis has been used and misused for many centuries. The stalks were harvested for rope (hence the term *hemp*) and cloth, the seeds for food, the flowers and leaves for both folk medicine and recreational intoxication.

Cannabis Compounds

It is important to note that a cannabis plant is polypharmaceutical—it contains hundreds and

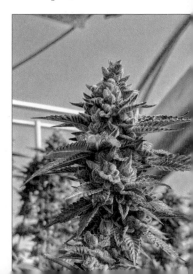

RIGHT: **The marijuana plant contains hundreds of different compounds. (photo credit: Steve Olson)**

hundreds of constituents, including a group called cannabinoids, some of which interact with other drugs by diminishing or accentuating effects of other nonprescription and prescription drugs.

Trichomes (glands) in the flower or bud of the marijuana plant contain dozens of different compounds that are collectively called cannabinoids. Tetrahydrocannabinol (THC) is a psychoactive cannabinoid. Hashish and hashish oil are the most intense extracts. Cannabidiol (CBD), cannabinol (CBN), cannabigerol (CBG), cannabichromene, and tetrahydrocannabivarin are cannabinoids that may provide relief for some cancer, seizure, or anxiety patients, or those suffering from inflammation, such as an animal with osteoarthritis. Additional names encountered for medical cannabis products are: tetrahydrocannabiniolic acid (THCA, depicted with or without a preceding delta or Δ), Δ-THC, and cannabidiolic acid (CBDA). The cannabis plant also contains the terpenoids (see *essential oils* for more on terpenes and terpenoids) β-caryophyllene, limonene, myrcene, and pinene.

Most cannabinoid products contain multiple cannabinoids, thus some percent of psychoactive THC is generally present in, for example, a CBD product that is primarily intended to reduce inflammation. There are many trade names for cannabinoid products intended for humans, and multiple companies manufacture cannabinoid products intended for animals, too.

Regulation

In 2018, Canada became the second country (Uruguay was the first) to fully legalize the possession, sale, and cultivation of marijuana. It is a myth that cannabis and CBD products are legal in many European countries; possession is illegal in Denmark, for example, although the act is often tolerated and prosecution is uncommon.

In the United States, federal law has long classified cannabis under schedule I, indicating it has a high potential for abuse and no known medical benefit. Thus, marijuana and its products remain largely illegal under US federal law as of 2020. However, the 2018 US Farm Bill, also called the Agricultural Improvement Act,

RIGHT: **Cannabis products, like all supplements, vary in how reliably they contain what the manufacturer advertises.**

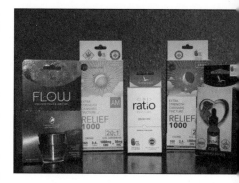

de-scheduled some cannabinoid products and allowed for low-THC hemp farming in some states, yet there are remaining conflicts with federal law. The Drug Enforcement Agency (DEA) is tasked with enforcing federal law and the Department of Agriculture (USDA) limits industrial cultivation of hemp. The Food and Drug Administration (FDA) recognized no medical benefit to cannabis products until very recently approving some CBD products for administration to some seizure patients. CBD and other cannabinoid products containing less than 0.003% THC are generally available through online purchase to all fifty states, although some states (Idaho, Nebraska, and South Dakota, as of 2019) still outlaw any cannabinoid.

Between 2015 and early 2019, the FDA issued forty-eight warning letters to a variety of companies selling various CBD, THC, and other cannabinoid products for a variety of offenses, including having *no cannabinoid in the product*. The FDA has also issued warnings to more than one company regarding marketing practices that included labeling their CBD products to be used in the prevention, mitigation, or treatment of disease in animals—an assertion that had not been proven in a clinical setting with standardized testing (large sample, randomized, double-blind, and reproducible studies).

Some states where marijuana remains illegal for recreational use do allow medicinal marijuana with a medical doctor's prescription for a human patient, but no states allow veterinarians to prescribe cannabis products for use in animals. Individual states receiving notice that a veterinarian suggested CBD could initiate an investigation.

About half of the states have decriminalized or legalized the products, thus enabling adult pet owners in those states to easily purchase CBD products at specific dispensaries within their state. In states where marijuana is not legal except for those with a medical marijuana card, that person may purchase cannabinoid products to administer to an animal.

Medical Application

Pain, anxiety, seizures, and poor appetite are legitimate problems for which some people have attempted to treat their animals with CBD and other cannabinoid products, with mixed results.

Cannabinoid products may be administered to an animal topically, such as rubbing CBD oil or gel on a sore joint, or more commonly as a supplement, such as a few drops of tincture added to the pet's food or dropped into the back of the mouth, an aerosol spray squirted on the tongue or gums, or a suppository inserted in the rectum. The cannabinoid is often in an oil form, with food-grade avocado oil or olive oil frequently being the base oil.

Veterinary practice is divided on the use of CBD for animals, with some alternative practitioners supporting and even manufacturing CBD products, while others cautioning that no large, well-designed studies have demonstrated cannabinoid efficacy for any ailment.

At least one small well-controlled study showed that dogs with osteoarthritis appeared (to both the study veterinarians and the dogs' owners) to become more active and more comfortable while being treated with at least two milligrams per kilogram of CBD twice per day (2 mg/kg BID). This was a double-blind study—neither the veterinarians nor the dog owners knew at the time whether the individual dog was receiving a placebo or the hemp oil product. And certainly, bacon-flavored cannabinoid compounds have eased more than one cancer-stricken pet to a more peaceful end.

Cautions

As noted above, the cannabis industry is not well monitored with regard to oversight that ensures a commercial product actually contains the cannabinoid advertised, or that it contains the amount the label asserts. Further, there is no oversight to ensure that a product does not also contain undesirable constituents, which means owners may unintentionally dose their pets with THC when attempting to relieve its pain or anxiety with CBD.

An animal's intoxication from THC may present as incontinence (loss of bladder control), vomiting, ataxia (staggering or uncoordinated gait), and muscle tremors. In US states that have legalized cannabis, animal emergency rooms have seen a marked uptick in patients—usually dogs—suffering ill effects from THC exposure and ingestion. Often these are accidental exposures. More than one dog has died from aspirating and choking on its own vomit after consuming a person's marijuana edibles. Sometimes, these exposures are recreational, the result of someone trying to get the animal high, intended as a prank or to gratify the person's curiosity about what would happen if the pet were intoxicated. Such an exposure is animal abuse, just as it is when a person intentionally gets an animal drunk on alcoholic beverages.

CHELATION THERAPY

Intravenous administration of a chelating agent is the conventional treatment for heavy metal poisoning. Cadmium and mercury are examples of these metals with a specific gravity greater than about 5.0. At the molecular level, there is a clawlike composition in the common chelating agent, ethylenediaminetetraacetic acid, also called *EDTA* or *edetic acid*. The Greek word for claw, *chele*, gives this therapy its name as EDTA binds metallic ions in the body in a stable form that is excreted in the urine. Calcium disodium EDTA is a chelating agent recommended for animals with lead poisoning. Chelation therapy has been extended to the alternative treatment sphere by practitioners who assert it helps in the treatment of vascular disease as well as other ailments.

The treatment is not without risks, as the chelating occurs not just in target ions, but in all ions to which the chelating agent has a molecular affinity. Thus zinc, copper, and calcium may also be flushed away. Further, the treatment has additional significant side effects.

Oral chelation therapy is also promoted by some practitioners and vendors of supplements as a treatment for geriatric confusion, which practitioners blame on aluminum toxicity. Like all supplements, they are not to be given without professional consultation.

COLLOIDAL MINERALS

A colloid is a substance composed of small particles suspended in another medium. For example, wood smoke from a campfire is a colloidal mix of solid soot particles suspended in gas. A hydrocolloid is composed of solid particles suspended in a liquid. Products marketed as colloidal minerals are liquid supplements with small mineral-containing particles suspended in water. There is a legend that colloidal minerals were accidentally discovered in the early 1900s by a rancher named Thomas Jefferson Parker who traced a Utah spring with reputed healing powers to their source and then mined the shale he found at the source to produce colloidal mineral water.

A veterinarian began promoting colloidal minerals as a treatment for numerous maladies and the tonic needed to secure perfect health. There are now numerous companies—many offering multilevel-marketing distributorships—selling colloidal minerals. Promotional literature for mines leaching minerals from rock shale out of Emery County, Utah, asserts that colloidal minerals are more complete and/or more absorbable by the body than mineral supplements in tablet form. One proponent asserts that long-lived cultures live near cold water enriched by glacially crushed rock, and the resultant *glacial milk* they drink is related to the peoples' longevity.

Predictably, some pet care retailers offer expensive (usually yellow-tinged) colloidal mineral supplements to pet owners. The majority of the periodic table of the elements is represented on some of the product labels, with the companies asserting that all of the elements are needed in supplemental form and all are necessary for optimum health. Consumers can balance those assertions with the knowledge that arsenic and lead, for example, are also naturally occurring elements in the earth's crust. The presence of an element on the planet does not equate to a mammal's need for supplementation of the element, even at trace levels.

COLLOIDAL SILVER

Following on the heels of the colloidal mineral interest is the promotion of colloidal silver, a liquid containing silver particles promoted as an ingestible health tonic or applied on wounds, rashes, and more. These products are sometimes created by electrically charging water in which a silver bar is submerged. Proponents correctly point out two advantages of colloidal silver over oral pharmaceutical antibiotics: bacteria do not seem to become resistant to silver, and ingested silver does not seem to cause dysbiosis (disruption of healthy gut bacteria).

However, while silver is known to have some antibacterial properties and has long been used topically in small amounts—such as in silver-impregnated bandages, especially for burn patients—there is no solid data to show that ingesting silver is beneficial.

A side effect of ingesting colloidal silver is *argyria*, a permanent discoloration of the skin to a bluish-gray hue. It is likely that the silver deposited in the skin is also deposited internally, in other body tissues. An Australian review and a separate study by an herbalist found that the risk of ingesting colloidal silver outweighs any possible benefit.

DIATOMACEOUS EARTH

Diatomaceous earth, also known as DE or diatomite, is a type of naturally occurring silica rock that is porous and abrasive. It is used industrially as an absorbent, filter, insulator, or as an insecticide. While the absorbent trait has led to its being used in the animal care world as kitty litter, its use as an insecticide has also brought DE into animal care, usually in the equine sphere. Crumbled into a powder, diatomaceous earth absorbs parts of the waxy outer layer of pests, bugs, and insects. The damage inflicted to the pests' bodies causes them to die prematurely.

As such, DE is used as a pest deterrent in settings such as grain storage. When mixed with an insect attractant, so that the pest will enter the diatomaceous earth powder, thus coating its body in DE, it becomes an insecticide.

Some people administer food-grade diatomaceous earth orally to wormy horses or dogs, although this is not an approved use of the product. Proponents note the worms cannot build up a tolerance to DE, as they can to chemical wormers, so rotation of worming preparations is unnecessary; but they must feed diatomaceous earth to the animal subject for a protracted period, often two to three months, in order to eradicate worms.

However, because diatomaceous earth is an absorbent, it loses its efficacy rapidly in a wet environment, and of course, an animal's digestive system is a wet environment.

Side effects of DE administration to animals can include weakening of the stomach wall and internal bleeding.

ESSENTIAL OILS

Essential oils (EOs) have long been used as perfumes and in cooking, as well as in folk medicine. Proponents sometimes point to the hundreds of times essential oils are mentioned in the old and new testaments as support for EO use in medical applications.

Frankincense, a sap derived from four varieties of the deciduous Boswellia shrub or tree (*Boswellia sacra*, *Boswellia frereana*, *Boswellia papyrifera*, and *Boswellia serrata*) has certainly been used in folk medicine throughout Asia, Africa, and Arabia since ancient times, as has myrrh, derived from the shrub *Commiphora*. Pliny the Elder, the Roman philosopher and naturalist, suggested myrrh and frankincense as antidotes to poisoning. Hippocrates suggested recipes that included myrrh, ox gall, honey, wine, saffron, pomegranate rind, frankincense, and lotus, with specific recommendations about when to mix the substances in a copper pot and when to place them in a bronze pot.

Essential oils are distilled from plants, often flowers which have glands called trichomes. The trichomes contain compounds called terpenes, which in turn release terpenoids that give the plant its distinctive scent and flavor. EOs are classed as volatile oils, meaning that they readily vaporize.

Essential oils are the mainstay of aromatherapy (see *Aromatherapy*). Many practitioners use EOs in a diffuser, which releases a very fine mist into the air. Others apply drops to surfaces in the home, kennel, cattery, barn, etc. while intending the EO to work as an inhalant. Still others apply the oils, usually diluted, directly onto an animal, intending the oil to penetrate the skin and be absorbed into the animal's body, and a few practitioners suggest ingestion of very specific EOs.

There exists an astounding range regarding which oils different practitioners suggest for various maladies, and many oils are blended together, such that there is an almost infinite list of different EOs. Practitioners who use EOs directly on the skin may rub the oils in circles and incorporate reflexology or other therapies (see *Reflexology* and *Vita Flex*) into the practice. Some practitioners believe that essential oils contain electromagnetic properties, while others attribute no magnetic properties to EO therapy.

There exists a schism in the practice of EOs between the majority who suggest always diluting the EO, and others who use undiluted EOs on animals. It is always safest to do a skin sensitivity test patch before applying even a diluted EO.

The American Kennel Club (AKC) warns dog owners that essential oils can be irritating to the dog's skin, and that an essential oil on the fur or skin may be licked off, thus accidentally ingested internally. (Note that this may be true for any animal.) The AKC further warns that essential oils of cinnamon, citrus, pennyroyal, peppermint, pine, sweet birch, tea tree (melaleuca), wintergreen, and ylang-ylang are outright toxic to dogs even when only applied topically.

The American Society for the Prevention of Cruelty to Animals (ASPCA) warns that cats are especially sensitive to essential oils and can be negatively affected by oils placed in a diffuser. The ASPCA cautions pet owners to not place an EO diffuser in the same room as their pet and not to run diffusers continuously. Animals exhibiting an initial overexposure to essential oils may drool, sneeze, cough, or vomit.

In addition to identifying what we know, it is important to recognize what we don't know. We don't know every EO that may be an endocrine disruptor. An endocrine disruptor is a chemical, constituent, or product that has the unintended side effect of disrupting a mammal's natural endocrine function, often by mimicking or interfering with a natural hormone. Early-onset puberty, low fertility, or different sex characteristics can be caused by endocrine disruption. We tend to think of endocrine disruption as brought on by excessive hormones fed to animals that are in our food chain, or caused by chemicals such as the phthalates in some nail polishes or otherwise in the environment through various products, but essential oils of lavender and tea tree have been implicated as endocrine disruptors, and other EOs remain poorly studied.

Those interested in learning more will encounter two organizations: The National Association of Aromatherapy and The Center for Aromatherapy Research and Education (CARE Inc.). CARE Incorporated is actually just run by one multilevel-marketing company that sells proprietary essential oils (see *Raindrop Technique*).

FLOWER ESSENCES

The usual understanding of the term *essence* as a distilled or concentrated extract would lead someone astray when examining flower essences. Here, flower essences are termed by some to be a vibrational therapy, in which a flower placed in a glass of water releases a vibration or energy into the water. The water is then used as a tonic. An extension of Edward Bach's original thirty-nine flower remedies, flower essences incorporate flowers Bach did not use as remedies as well as combinations and flowers that he did claim for a specific complaint.

GLANDULAR THERAPY

Treating disease through the administration of another animal's gland, or preparations prepared from harvested glands, is an ancient practice. The treatment springs from the belief that a supplement made from an eyeball will help an eye problem and so on.

Oral tolerization, feeding small but often increasing doses, has been experimented with in both conventional and alternative circles with interesting results that give hope, especially for certain autoimmune disorders.

There is concern regarding the source material for these products. Thousands of bears are currently in captivity for harvesting products from them, for example, their bile. Some practitioners consider the bear to be a walking pharmacy.

Glandular therapy is related to *cell therapy*, in which practitioners administer—orally or via injection—freeze-dried or fresh cells from another organism to a patient. This is also called *live cell* therapy by some practitioners and is often confused with *stem cell therapy* (which is also called cell therapy), an emerging field of mainstream medicine that uses stem cells, although there are some applications of stem cells that are not approved—not proven to be effective—and thus are properly termed alternative treatments.

Live cell therapy, or cell therapy, applies harvested, mature donor cells. It has not been conclusively proven to be of value to the patient. The issue can be confusing for consumers because proponents of cell therapy may promote administration of embryonic cells. Again, these embryo cells are not stem cells, in the histological sense. They are mature cells from an embryo and an alternative treatment, apart from modern stem cell science.

HOMEOPATHY

Homeopathic remedies are a very highly diluted form of herbs and other preparations.

See the therapists section, *What Is a Homeopath?*

HOMOTOXICOLOGY

In the late 1920s, Hans-Heinrich Reckeweg, a German physician with an interest in homeopathy, developed the theory of homotoxicology, that disease was caused by endogenous (within the body) or exogenous (external to the body) toxins or homotoxins. In contrast with classical homeopathy, which suggests only one remedy is to be administered at a time, homotoxicology often combines multiple preparations and may use less diluted preparations.

Reckeweg published a text on homotoxicology in 1955 and relocated to Albuquerque, New Mexico, in the late 1970s, forming a company called Biological Homeopathic Industries, now known as HEEL (for the latin, *herba est ex luce*, meaning "plants come from light"), to market the remedies. As may have been expected, his work was adopted by numerous animal practitioners. In 1984, he was warned by the FDA that his anticancer potions were not known to be safe and effective.

MEGAVITAMIN THERAPY

Distinct from orthomolecular medicine only in its concentration on vitamins, megavitamin therapy is still often used synonymously with both orthomolecular medicine and augmentation therapy.

The world's demand for vitamins that are added to processed foods, including commercial pet food, or vitamins available as supplements—including the supplements used for megavitamin therapy— is satisfied via synthesis. Although vitamins are natural substances, they are synthesized from surprisingly industrial sources.

Acetone and formaldehyde are two of the ingredients that go into the manufacturing of vitamin A. A leftover waste product from the manufacturing of nylon is used to make niacin (vitamin B3). Vitamin C is created in a multistep process that involves bacteria fermenting the sugar alcohol sorbitol into sorbose. Next, a genetically modified bacteria ferments the sorbose in 2-ketogluconic acid. Hydrochloric acid turns the 2-ketogluconic acid into ascorbic acid, otherwise known as vitamin C. Vitamin D is synthesized by irradiating and chemically treating lanolin (the natural oil in sheep wool) to create cholecalciferol, which is another name for vitamin D. Chemicals extracted from coal tar go into the manufacture of thiamin (vitamin B1).

While these industrial processes may be surprising and unnatural, they are not inherently unhealthy, but rather are accepted manufacturing realities. But this information should highlight why it is good to acquire vitamins through daily good nutrition rather than through supplementation.

Note that some vitamins are fat soluble (vitamins A, D, E, and K), allowing them to build to toxic levels in the body, while others are water soluble, so excess is much more easily excreted. Thus, as with all supplements and other treatments, do not casually administer them.

By convention, some B vitamins are more commonly called by their chemical names while others are known by a letter and number. The B vitamins are listed here for clarity:

B_1	thiamine
B_2	riboflavin
B_3	niacin
B_5	pantothenic acid
B_6	pyrodoxine
B_7	biotin
B_9	folic acid
B_{12}	cobalamin

NOSODES

Joseph Wilhelm Lux, a veterinarian homeopath who practiced in the 1830s, suggested *isopathy* for disease prevention—treating a disease with the disease agent. Thus nosodes are born, the homeopathic answer to vaccination. A pathological specimen, such as diseased tissue, saliva, pus, or other discharge, is diluted to homeopathic proportions and administered orally to the animal. See the therapists section—*What Is a Homeopath?*—to appreciate this dilution.

The consensus of the veterinary community at large, even among the majority of alternative practice veterinarians researched for this book, is that nosodes do not offer the protection from disease that vaccination does. Any treatment at homeopathic dilution contains nothing but the dilutant.

Concurrent with the interest in nosodes is a general anti-vaccine, or anti-unnecessary-vaccine movement. The former ignores the tremendous benefits vaccination has conferred on animals, while the latter has some merit. As such, vaccine recommendations for animals have been revised for some species, in some areas, regarding some diseases. That said, owners who simply refuse all vaccines (often in fear of an unspecified post-vaccine illness sometimes called vaccinosis) place not only their own animals at great risk, but other animals as well as the human population.

NUTRACEUTICALS

Nutraceutical is a relatively new term for substances that are not drugs (and so are not subject to federal regulation, review, and efficacy in the United States) but are rather foods or food parts intended to give health benefits. They are not necessarily herb preparations either, although they can be. Glucosamine and chondroitin, commonly given for joint complaints (although their efficacy is still debated), are examples of nutraceuticals. Like many terms, there is more than one definition for *nutraceutical*. Health Canada, the Canadian office assigned federal responsibility for human health, narrows the meaning to "preparations" that are not strictly foods and are "*demonstrated to promote health or prevent disease.*"

In the United States, products classified as nutraceuticals have a variable track record of actually containing the substance claimed on the packaging.

NUTRITION THERAPY

Diet is certainly one of the greatest single influences on health, and manipulation of an animal's diet is a sure way to impact its well-being. While people will debate the pros and cons between home-cooked, natural, Bones and Raw Food (BARF), or commercially prepared pet food—and the dog food industry suffered an enormous black eye with the 2007 melamine contamination problem—the simplest and surest view of dietary requirements remains one of common sense, in which the animal receives essential nutrition of good quality.

Nutrition therapy as a special therapeutic treatment, however, aims to exert a greater influence over health, for instance by anticipating additional requirements due to impending stress, such as surgery, moving, or competition, and is recognized by the American Holistic Veterinary Medical Association as a separate modality. Nutrition therapy remains a strong component of TCVM as well.

Probiotics—a microbial supplement believed to enhance the animal's natural, healthy intestinal flora—are an example of a common nutritional recommendation. The results of many studies on probiotics are mixed. It is recognized that gut flora from one species often do not transfer or colonize successfully in another species. Also, see the segment on herbalism for a warning about cross-species errors, such as alliums in canine diets. Prebiotics are meant to provide nourishment for the desirable microbes. We now know that an animal's gut bacteria generally changes very little throughout its life, thus neither prebiotics nor probiotics produce much effect on the microbiome.

ORTHOMOLECULAR MEDICINE

In the 1950s, Nobel laureate Linus Pauling developed the concept of *orthomolecular* (literally, the *right molecule*) medicine with an initial application in human psychiatry that soon spread to general health. He advocated significantly higher doses of certain vitamins than was, and is, commonly accepted by the medical community. Veterinary orthomolecular medicine is today a specialty of some holistic practitioners who suggest high-dose administration of vitamins, minerals, amino acids, and other supplements to a specific animal in a specific set of circumstances. Its hallmark is that there is not one set of recommendations for all animals of a species, but rather, the recommendations are based on individual need.

PHEROMONE THERAPY

A pheromone is a chemical an animal naturally produces and releases to communicate with other animals. Pheromone therapy, also called pheromonotherapy, attempts to exploit the effect of pheromones in behavioral or training situations.

When a cat rubs its temples and whiskers on another cat or another animal, including a human, the chemical released is called feline facial pheromone; when synthesized, it is called feline facial pheromone analogue (FFPA). Another example of a pheromone is the chemical alpha-casozepine, which lactating mares release near their mammary glands; the chemical calms the nursing foal. Alpha-casozepine has been synthesized and called Equine Appeasing Pheromone (EAP). Predictably, there is a product for canines called Dog Appeasing Pheromone (DAP), and a product for calming cats.

Pheromone therapy products are available as sprays, wipes, or atomizers.

Well-designed studies have yielded mixed results in which the practitioners did not know until after the animals had been treated, studied, and scored whether the subject animal had been given a placebo or the genuine pheromone product. A 2015 study (Conti, et al) of thirty cats tested at home and in a veterinary hospital showed no difference between treated and untreated cats with regard to their reactivity, blood pressure, heart rate, and other parameters.

A double-blind study of forty horses that were placed in an unusual and potentially fear-inducing situation (being made to walk through a fringed curtain) found the horses that were treated with EAP had significantly lower heart rates and better cooperation than horses treated with placebo. In a small study of six semi-feral ponies, the treated ponies were found to be gentler than those treated with a placebo. A study of fourteen foals who were abruptly weaned found no difference between treated and untreated foals in their stress hormone (cortisol) release, or the stress-related behavior. A systematic review of fourteen studies that used pheromones on dogs and cats found insufficient evidence of effectiveness of DAP and FFPA.

TRADITIONAL CHINESE VETERINARY MEDICINE

TCM/TCVM focuses strongly on acupuncture, tui na, qigong, nutrition therapy, and herbalism. Eastern herbs are frequently prescribed as tea pills—small black pills that can be administered directly although they were meant to be dissolved in water and taken as a tea. The organic materials used in TCVM include *dilong* (earthworm), dozens of herbs, plant combinations, and more. True practitioners place great emphasis on proper diagnosis under the rubric of their schooling, which includes believing in an effect on a body by five elements (earth, wood, water, metal, wind), the four seasons, and more. Concepts of wind invasion, dryness, and dampness are studied and impact treatment recommendations. Practitioners are taught that things have a complementary yin to the yang. Meats that are believed to be inherently hot (venison, lamb, chicken) are fed for what are believed to be cold conditions, while protein believed to be cold (rabbit, duck, turkey, white fish, clams) are fed to animals with what are viewed as hot conditions.

Believed by many practitioners to be a whole medical system, TCVM is sometimes combined with conventional medicine, though with difficulty given the different views of causation of disease.

Warning: it is impossible to ethically discuss TCVM without addressing the existence of bile bears and other wildlife abuses. Throughout numerous countries (China, Laos, Myanmar, South Korea, Vietnam), more than ten thousand bears are kept for their entire lives in cages the size of coffins for the purpose of extracting bile from the bears' gallbladders twice per day. The coveted substance in bear bile is called ursodiol or ursodeoxycholic acid (USDA) and it is used, among other things, to treat gallstones. Ursodiol can be synthesized in a laboratory, but in some locales in Asia, it is harvested from the bile bears to be used in the production of some TCVM remedies. Sometimes the live bile bears' feet are amputated so that their paws can be used in remedies.

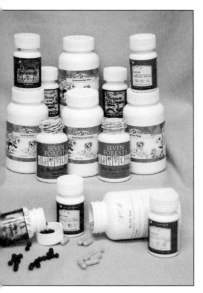

LEFT: **Tea pills are a mainstay of Chinese herbalism.**

Other wildlife body parts such as tiger bones, rhino horn, tortoiseshell, and animal teeth are used in other folk remedies. These wildlife body parts are illegal to possess in many Western countries, yet people purchasing TCVM services may be unaware of the industry they are supporting when they become part of the market by purchasing proprietary remedies made of undisclosed constituents. Even if the remedies an alternative practitioner uses do not have illicit ingredients, if the manufacturer is in business with the bile bear industry, then any purchases from that vendor support that ugly business.

The sight of a warehouse of bears, each in a cage so tight it cannot turn around, moaning in their miserable existence, their cries heightened as metal catheters puncture their abdomens and then their gall bladders to drain bile is horrifying—and one this author will not again subject herself to—but nonetheless it is a sight that every person interested in TCVM ought to view.

TISSUE SALTS

Wilhelm Heinrich Schüssler, a homeopath who practiced in the 1800s, developed the concept that mineral salt imbalances caused physical or behavioral problems. He thought many conditions could be remedied with minute doses of one or more of these twelve salts:

Also called *biochemic tissue salts* or *cell salts*, the salts are not technically a homeopathic remedy because they do not operate on homeopathy's founding principle of "Like Cures Like" although they are diluted to homeopathic levels. See the therapists section—*What Is a Homeopath?*—to understand this dilution.

Schüssler's Salts
calcium fluoride
calcium phosphate
calcium sulphate
ferric phosphate
magnesium phosphate
potassium chloride
potassium phosphate
potassium sulphate
silicon dioxide
sodium chloride
sodium phosphate
sodium sulphate

A combination of all twelve remedies is called *Bioplasma*. Tissue salts are sometimes recommended by naturopaths and homeopaths for a range of allergic, inflammatory, respiratory, and neurological problems in addition to emotional trauma. Some advocates of tissue salt treatment identify a correlation between Schüssler's twelve salts and the twelve zodiac signs. Conventional veterinarians and other scientists recognize that the highly diluted doses in the prepared remedies are far too small to impact body chemistry, so attribute any success of their administration to the placebo effect.

UROTHERAPY

Urotherapy, also called urine therapy, is the practice of treating the animal with urine, either through ingestion (having the animal drink urine or adding it to the animal's food) or topically (such as applying the urine to the animal's gums, or soaking its foot). When the animal's own urine is collected and used as the supplement, the practice is called auto-urine therapy, but donated urine may be used in urotherapy.

A veterinarian whose practice centers strongly on alternative treatments asserts that urotherapy helps alleviate seizures, allergies, and electrolyte imbalances, among other ailments.

It is true that ingesting one's own urine is an ancient practice, and it is true that urine is sterile, but remember that urine is a waste product, like feces, and the body is excreting it for a number of reasons.

There is no scientific evidence to support rinsing an animal in urine or making it consume urine, no matter whether the urine is collected from the animal patient or is donated from another animal.

WATER

Altered water or water that is purported to be altered or improved via the addition of special drops or the application of special devices is often sold—or the drops or devices are sold—as a general health tonic to be used as general drinking water and/or applied topically.

These alterations or attempted modifications to water include: acidified water, activated water, alkaline water, bound water, catalytic water treatment, clustered water, energized water, exploded water, far infrared (FIR) treated water, fractal water, hexagonal water, hydrogen-bonded water, inducted water, ionized water, Kangen water, magnet-treated water, micro-clustered water, oxygenated water, pentagonal water, reduced water, structured water, super-ionized water, vitalized water, vortex-treated water, zeta potential water. An excellent site to review water chemistry and quackery is www.chem1.com.

The sales pitches for altered (or supposedly altered) waters generally promise improved hydration due to the reputedly improved water. These advertised improvements often subvert science. For example, clusters and hexagonal or pentagonal chains of water molecules actually last for mere picoseconds (trillionths of a second); oxygen added to water is rapidly released into the atmosphere, and ingested oxygen cannot improve tissue oxygenation in mammals. In other cases, these advertised improvements to water depend upon mystical beliefs (energizing or vitalization).

The basic chemistry of water is two hydrogen atoms and one oxygen atom making one molecule of water. Water molecules are in constant motion and do swap bonds between hydrogen ions, briefly changing, for example, the pH, thus making some of the water more acid or more alkaline; but these extremely brief chemical changes do not last. Water is known to pass through cell membranes one molecule at a time, and there is no such thing as a smaller shape of water than a single molecule. In any case, modifications to basic, clean drinking water are unnecessary.

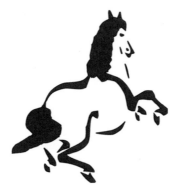

Mystical Therapies

SCIENCE-BASED PROFESSIONALS MAY argue that perhaps all alternative treatments should be classified under the realm of the mystical, and they will be making a fair argument because the treatments rest on belief. However, if one is seeking measurable, reproducible results that will withstand significant scientific testing, then one is not seeking alternative treatments at all.

Metaphysical claims are inherently unable to be proved, so compatible belief systems are a requirement for mystical therapies. Many of these treatments are also referred to as *energy healing* or *vibrational therapy* (although there is not a commonly accepted, specific definition for either of these terms).

There are essentially no side effects with mystical treatments, but skeptics point to a reasonable concern that competent care can be displaced by attention to alternative efforts.

ASTROLOGY

Horoscope readings for animals are done by many practitioners who work on people. The practice can be used by clients who are seeking guidance in making decisions about their animals, including their health. Using the zodiac signs, stars, and planets for specific guidance is an ancient practice that worked well for mariners, but people have long looked to the sky for answers to ambiguous questions too. There are practitioners who claim to divine help for example, on whether or not to show or train or breed an animal, based upon the positions of celestial bodies.

AURA ADJUSTMENT

Believers feel an aura—similar to an atmosphere or energy field—surrounds living things, and some people are sensitive enough to read this aura. The aura can then be interpreted and possibly adjusted.

CHAKRA ADJUSTMENT

Chakra is a Sanskrit word referring to a wheel, circle, or center. The chakra concept holds that there are seven points of energy concentration along the body's central nervous system. Extended to colors and seven types of tissue, the concept of chakras is rooted in ayurvedic medicine, including veterinary practice, although there are new interpretations of the belief that are more New Age than ancient.

Other chakra charts enumerate eight different chakras. One equine chakra chart of seven points (brow, crown, throat, heart, solar plexus, sacrum, and root) identifies seven elements said to correspond to a horse's chakra points: silver, gold, ether, air, fire, water, and earth.

Color therapy is one area that often combines a belief in chakras, choosing corresponding colors in an attempt to adjust an animal.

A *mandala* (Sanskrit reference to circle or completion, but in the alternative treatment and artistic circles referring to a diagram or drawing imbued with significance, like a geometric Navajo sand painting or many Asian cultures' design offerings) figure often accompanies chakra work, as may the use of crystals. Still other practitioners offer an array of touch, supplementation, mystical, and other services all under the heading of balancing the animal's chakra.

CHI/JI/KI/QI ADJUSTMENT

Believers view chi (and the various permutations of its spelling when transliterated into English) as the vital force in a living being. Practitioners believe they can assess and possibly adjust the chi. While most practitioners hail from the TCVM branch of alternative treatments, some offer qi adjustment services independently of any other training or belief system.

CRYSTALS

Crystal healing is an old practice that seems to have grown almost wherever crystals were encountered by the indigenous peoples. The rocks (and resin, in the form of amber) are credited with various strengths or capacities relating to the body and are usually simply placed near the animal being treated. Some practitioners use crystal necklaces on horses in an effort to make them more amenable to training. Tourmaline crystals are sometimes placed in water in the hope of improving water quality.

Other practitioners administer ground crystals or minerals in an animal's food or water—such a remedy may be marketed as a *gem elixir*—and would be classified as a supplemental treatment.

Bird of No Paradise

Caged birds aren't living their natural life, but no animal absorbed into common human living situations—no pet—is.

One particular parrot had been known to be a bad bird. To bite. She also became exorbitantly stressed about small changes in the household, company visiting or an object moved. Worse, when the bird was less than perky and its owners consulted a veterinarian who specialized in avian medicine, they were frightened by his matter-of-fact comment that by the time a sick bird is brought to a vet, it is often too late.

"In the wild, it is not in the bird's best interest to look sick," he added. "It will be the next one hunted if it looks weak. Birds are amazing about seeming OK until they are just about to drop dead."

Could there be a light at the end of the tunnel for a bad bird who sometimes got a bit down?

Actually, lights, in the form of both color therapy and heliotherapy, were recommended by one animal wellness practitioner. An alternative veterinarian said crystals were the answer.

She recommended placing a quartz crystal in all birds' water bowls or water bottles to energize the water. She believes crystals impart a strengthening energy that helps birds be resistant to, and recover from, avian diseases as well as common mites and other parasites. She urges people to not think of animals as only physical beings and asserts that sickness occurs when the life force is

LEFT: **Could the crystal in this parrot's water improve its health?**

weakened. Crystals help the life force stay strong, she advised.

"I wonder if you have to believe in it for it to work," the owner said.

The alternative vet sold expensive crystals, as well as a variety of homeopathic formulas of her own making and nutritional supplements.

The owner placed a three-dollar quartz crystal from a rock shop (the store proprietor advised the crystal he sold had good energy) in the bird's water and waited for results.

The parrot calmed down over time, became more social—a good bird. However, the owner could not attribute the improved behavior to the rock in the water.

DETOXIFICATION THERAPY

Detoxification means different things to different therapists. Many products are sold under the heading of detoxification treatments, including oral herbal formulas that are usually intended to serve as gastrointestinal or hepatic (liver) cleanses, products intended to be used as colonics or enemas (sometimes classified as a form of hydrotherapy and termed *entero-hydrotherapy*) and electric machines that are intended to detoxify the patient (one electric detoxification unit has a coil that is immersed in a basin of water with the patient's foot).

Because detoxification has become a buzzword, it is important to clarify what a practitioner means when detoxification therapy is advocated. Often, practitioners are unable to specify what toxins they claim to be removing from an animal in the detoxification teatment.

If they assert that they are removing something vague, such as environmental pollutants, or slightly more specific, such as heavy metals, there is no measurement conducted that confirms the presence and then removal of the alleged toxin.

DOWSING AND PENDULUM ASSESSMENT

Dowsing, or assessment via pendulum swinging, is sometimes practiced with a crystal over the body in an attempt to discern the problem area, or even over a map to try to identify, for example, the location of a lost dog. Dowsing is also used to select a remedy, for example, swinging a pendulum by a selection of Bach flower essences or homeopathic remedies. While there are practitioners who claim success at dowsing and pendulum swinging, a British study (McCarney, et al) of six dowsing homeopaths had negative results—the homeopaths were less than 50 percent accurate in divining between a homeopathic remedy or a placebo.

FENG SHUI

Chinese for "wind-water," *feng shui* is the ancient practice of attempting to encourage positive chi through the best possible arrangement of a structure or other surroundings. A practitioner who offers feng shui services to pet owners may evaluate an owner's home and suggest a different-colored dog bed, or moving the cat's

BELOW: **Feng shui seeks to optimize chi in the animal's environment through careful selection and placement of objects.**

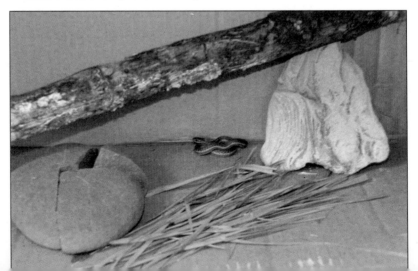

bowl to a specific area of the house. Practitioners may use mandalas when assessing feng shui and may offer specific changes when an animal is healing from an illness or injury.

HYPNOSIS

When Friedrich Anton (Franz) Mesmer, an Austrian physician born in 1734, spoke of animal magnetism, he coined the phrase with meanings of his time, invoking the idea of a tide-like force within all living human and other animal bodies. He treated patients with the use of magnets and calming gestures. France's King Louis XVI had a commission (composed of Benjamin Franklin, Jean Bailly, Antoine Lavoisier, and Joseph Guillotin) to investigate whether Mesmer had indeed discovered a new bodily force akin to magnetic pull. The commission decided that Mesmer had not made a legitimate discovery.

A by-product of Mesmer's work was the accidental invention of hypnosis. Today hypnosis practitioners for animals focus most work on behavioral disorders that contribute to health and training problems, without adding on a belief about animal magnetism.

PSYCHICS AND ANIMAL COMMUNICATORS

In addition to the encounter related earlier in this book (*Into the Mystic*) about a visit to a psychic, the author has interviewed others who have consulted a pet psychic and reported an experience that was helpful or amazing. Some communicators claim several levels of communication with animals, identified as clairvoyance (seeing), clairsentience (feeling or sensing), and clairaudience (channeling). One animal practitioner claims a mentor channels a saint. In this manner, multilevel communication practitioners report a variant of Gestalt practice (a human psychotherapy), which purports to allow the communicator to see the animal's perspective, specifically the animal's present perception. Communicators are found working in situations as diverse as behavioral problems, lost animals, and diagnostics—the latter being an effort to communicate with an animal about the ailment.

QIGONG

Some aspects of traditional Chinese veterinary medicine fall under the realm of mystical treatments because of the nature of belief regarding chi/ji/ki/qi. Those who believe in the concept of this life force, thought to regulate vital energy and blood flow, may also believe chi can be manipulated through *qigong* (or qi gong), *t'ai chi,* and *tui na.* Because this theoretical life force cannot be measured or identified, it is difficult to identify exactly how or when or if the force could be manipulated, but qigong takes the appearance of a combination of mystical treatment, with some motion and even touch added, depending upon the practitioner.

REIKI

Mikao Usui, born in Japan in 1865, is credited with being the founder of reiki (usually pronounced *ray-key*). It is a mystical treatment with a physical touching component. Some practitioners consider it a sacred healing art, and students are sometimes blindfolded when under instruction. Physically, it generally consists of gentle finger pressure in an effort to relieve pain or stress, but practitioners further believe they are channeling energy for health purposes, thus making reiki an example of a mystical treatment or energy medicine.

THERAPEUTIC TOUCH

Dolores Krieger, a nurse and professor emeritus of New York University's Division of Nursing, and Dora Kunz, a theosophist and president of the Theosophical Society in America from 1975 to 1987, introduced therapeutic touch in 1972. While nurses were the first practitioners and humans were the first patients, the practice spread to animal patients, with numbers of specialists now offering the treatment. Therapeutic touch must be classed as a mystical treatment because it is generally considered an energy treatment, not a physical action. In therapeutic touch, the practitioners often do not touch the animal, but rather hold their hands near the patient, attempting to release and alter energy fields around the animal's body in a

RIGHT: **Therapeutic Touch practitioners actually do not touch the animal during treatment.**

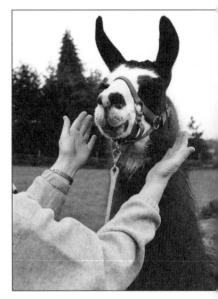

four-step process of centering, assessing, unruffling, and transferring energy.

In 1998, *the Journal of the American Medical Association* (*JAMA*) published a study conducted by Emily Rosa, a nine-year-old girl, in which twenty-one therapeutic touch practitioners, who asserted they would be able to detect a person's biofield, energy, or presence, were able to correctly identify a person's presence only 44 percent of the time. Mere guessing by an untrained person should have yielded a correct guess about 50 percent of the time. While Krieger countered the study's methodology, others supported the research debunking therapeutic touch.

THOUGHT FIELD THERAPY

Thought field therapy is a human psychological treatment that consists of verbal communication, with the patient concentrating on a specific problem, such as a fear of flying, and the practitioner then completing a series of finger taps on various points of the patient's body. In the United States and the United Kingdom, the practice has extended to animals. Practitioners report success in resolving behavioral problems, such as aggression or shying, after treatment.

VIBRATIONAL THERAPY

Many alternative practitioners use the term *vibrational* or *vibration therapies* either as a synonym for energy healing or as a collective term for the healing source for various alternative treatments.

This concept of vibration therapy differs from that of vibrating devices used in some animal rehabilitation facilities to stimulate circulation and tissue rebuilding. Pulsed electromagnetic field therapy, for example, creates a vibration that is imperceptible to people, but still present. Tuning forks create an easily perceptible vibration and may be referred to by some practitioners as a vibrational therapy. Numerous devices classified as vibration therapies are also called bioresonance therapies, and these are dealing with the concept of vibrational healing that is synonymous with energy healing or bioresonance.

Some practitioners offering *bioresonance* describe it as a testing procedure assessing what they view as the animal's *biofield,* a force they perceive to flow through or from the animal.

VITA FLEX

Vita Flex is a portmanteau of *vitality* through *reflexes.* Stanley Burroughs, also known as Aaron Hayes, is alternatively credited with developing Vita Flex or with bringing the theory from Tibet. He was better known for developing a diet for humans called the master cleanse, had no medical training, and was criminally charged with practicing medicine without a license. Predictably, Vita Flex therapy, which combines elements of essential oils and naturopathy with acupressure, reflexology and mystical belief, is also offered to animals.

Some of the practices of Vita Flex are incorporated into a more recently developed treatment called Raindrop Technique, but few remaining alternative care for animals practitioners offer strict Vita Flex practice. (See *Raindrop Technique*).

ZERO BALANCING

Zero balancing, sometimes hyphenated or abbreviated (zero-balancing, or ZB), is a therapy that combines the practitioner touching and thinking in an effort to use energy healing for the patient. It was started in the 1970s by Fritz Smith as a treatment for humans. Like many alternative treatments for people, it more recently crossed over into animal therapy. Practitioners use finger pressure and hold stretches while attempting to release energy.

Other Alternative Therapies

WHAT'S LEFT? WHILE some of the following therapies might have been classified as mystical due to their foundation on an unproven belief, another component of the treatment places them here. Alternative treatments that cannot be strictly classified as a touch, supplemental, or mystical therapy include more invasive treatments, such as acupuncture, larval therapy, and stem cells. Other therapies here are not invasive but still cannot be categorized strictly as a form of touch therapy, a supplement, or something that is necessarily mystical in scope, and others are classed in this category because they are whole systems, or merely diagnostic in effort.

While some of these other alternatives are invasive, most are not. Generally speaking, none have been widely accepted by the established scientific community as proven to improve a condition, but again, that is the hallmark of alternative treatments. Exceptions are larval therapy, which is proven but remains rare and is sometimes considered an alternative treatment, and treatments that are grounded in science, such as nutrigenomics and stem cell therapy, but are then applied in an ungrounded manner that pushes them into the realm of alternative treatments.

Side effects among these other therapies are variable, depending upon the therapy itself.

ACUPUNCTURE

See first the special earlier review of this subject. Modern animal acupuncturists may or may not use specific acupuncture points and may or may not follow the concept of meridians. In addition to the various manual and device methods (including the use of colored lights, a method known as *colorpuncture*, see also *esogetic colorpuncture*) of acupressure, acupuncture is expanded by those who perform it with topical or subdermal electrodes or needles to which electrodes are attached (*electro-acupuncture*).

Some acupuncturists rotate the needles during or after insertion, and claim that the rotation is key to activating or releasing qi.

Aquapuncture refers to the injection of liquid into acupressure points. The practitioner may use a vitamin solution, saline, or local anesthetic in an effort to increase the effect on the acupressure point.

While practitioners do not all agree about applications and devices, they also disagree on terminology. *Ting point therapy*, another variant on acupuncture, is described both as stimulation of the most distal points of an animal's digits, the paw or hoof, or as therapeutic stimulation of tendinomuscular meridians.

Another controversial therapy is the implantation of acupuncture material, usually *gold beads*, into the body. These implants have been shown to migrate and cause unintended, negative effects.

Only sterile, disposable needles should be used for acupuncture. Bruising is the most common side effect, and infection is always a possibility.

Aquapuncture: The Weal of Fortune

A subcutaneous (under the skin) injection forms a temporary weal, a small bump under the skin where the foreign fluid is deposited. An example of a weal being desirable is when a patient needs a large bore needle inserted. A practitioner might first use a very small needle to inject a small amount of anesthetic, such as lidocaine, under the skin to make a small weal exactly where she wishes to puncture the skin with the large needle. Now when she inserts the large needle (nail!) into the patient through the weal, it is painless.

Alternative practitioners have expanded acupuncture to aquapuncture. They create weals by injecting saline or vitamin solutions at sites where they wish to create an aquapuncture weal.

One veterinarian told me he doesn't practice dry needling (acupuncture) at all, but he does perform aquapuncture on his equine patients.

"I use a vitamin B_{12} solution. It doesn't really matter if you use a vitamin or a saline solution, but most horses are deficient in B_{12} anyway, so I use B_{12}."

This vet has not long been a practitioner of alternative treatments.

"I didn't believe in any of that voodoo," he told me. He learned the aquapuncture technique from another veterinarian.

"What happens is the weal keeps pressure on the acupuncture point longer, maintains the pressure for a while after I've left."

He reported using aquapuncture for a range of symptoms, but most commonly applies the therapy for pain relief to lame or stiff horses. He's been a veterinarian a long time and has seen countless patients in diverse situations—and in very similar circumstances. Because he's been in the field both before he ever used aquapuncture and since he incorporated the procedure in his practice, he's become a believer.

AROMATHERAPY

The idea that a pleasant scent can affect one's mood is easy to understand. However, people must remind themselves that animals generally have a far more acute sense of smell than humans do. An animal could be swamped in a scent that seems mildly pleasant to

BELOW: **Aromatherapy. Remember that animals have a keener sense of smell than people.**

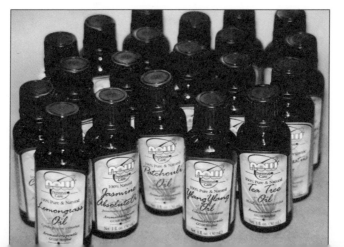

a person. Essential oils, usually used in aromatherapy, are distilled products that contain terpenes (organic compounds produced by plants) or terpoids (modified terpenes). Some aromatherapists suggest massaging a small amount of a an essential oil or other scented liquid onto an animal to aid in behavioral adjustment, while some would apply the scented oil or water to bedding or in an open container near the animal. Again, owners should be aware of the animal's more acute sense of smell.

AURAL PHOTOGRAPHY

In aural photography, standard film or digital photographic equipment is manipulated in an attempt to reveal the subject's aura. The manipulation may occur during photography (with the addition of fiber optics or adjustment to the light, time exposure, or lens focal length) or during film development, which in the case of digital aural photography employs digital enhancement or editing. Practitioners may attempt to diagnose disturbances in a subject's aura or to prove a treatment is working because of a difference between *before* and *after* aura photographs.

AYURVEDA

Ayurveda is a healing tradition from India that is considered by many to be a whole medical system. It has long been extended to practice on animals. An ancient text called *Aswa-ayurveda* detailed equine medicine. Ayurveda includes herbalism, Hindu philosophy, and a belief in an adjustable life force called the *prana* (akin to the Chinese belief in *qi*, or the ancient Greek belief in *pneuma*).

The body is viewed as a reflection of the earth with the five ayurvedic elements (earth, air, fire, water, and ether) corresponding to the five senses.

COLOR THERAPY

Color therapy, also called *chromotherapy,* makes good simple sense at its basic level. Who wouldn't avoid sitting in a room with black walls, and who wouldn't prefer a sunnier color? The idea that animals are strictly color-blind is likely a bit of an overstatement, just as is the notion that humans cannot see in the dark. True, animals' eyes generally have more rods (which work with light) than cones (which work with color) while humans have the reverse arrangement, but people do have rods and can see somewhat in the dark. It is likely that animals have some color perception.

Practitioners have developed attempts to influence animals' physical and mental behavior with color. Color therapy has evolved into an alternative treatment that incorporates different-colored lights that the animal is exposed to, and even to the use of water that has been exposed to different-colored lights. These treated waters are called *color essences*. The water is then sold in small spray bottles to be applied as desired. For example, water that was exposed to green light is sprayed inside a horse trailer in hope of calming a horse that is a poor traveler.

Color therapists often rely on ayurvedic tradition with the chakra concept and assign seven or eight colors to specific behavioral effects.

While there is a significant body of psychological studies on humans that demonstrates marked influence on human behavior due to the impact of color on our choices—such as Black Dog Syndrome, the name animal shelters give to the difficulty in getting black dogs adopted, thus more black-coated dogs are killed in shelters because potential adopters see them as more dangerous than light-colored dogs—conducting such studies on animals is problematic, and the research just isn't there to support color therapy.

CUPPING

Also known as fire cupping, the ancient practice involves creating a light suction on the body by means of a small heated cup that is inverted on the skin. Animals' fur can interfere with the creation of suction, so the practitioner may shave or gel the area to be cupped. Often numerous cups are used.

There is a risk of burns from the hot cup.

The health benefit is believed to be essentially restoring balance by drawing out whatever is believed to be in excess or relieving stagnation. Some practitioners restrict the practice to acupressure points.

Although cupping has been practiced on most continents and in numerous cultures (it is mentioned in an old Jewish proverb and a Muslim hadith as well as writings from Eastern Europe, Asia, and Mexico), it is most commonly associated with TCVM.

DARK FIELD MICROSCOPY

Günther Enderlein, a German zoologist, studied blood samples under dark field microscopy and published his findings in 1925. This method of microscopic study shows the image in reverse, like a negative. In the modern world of alternative treatments for animals, dark field microscopy (DFM), or *live blood analysis,* is an examination of a drop of the fasting pet's fresh blood under a microscope, without using a bright light to illuminate the slide holding the blood. Some practitioners believe they can determine more about a pet's health via DFM, and they choose a remedy such as polysan or Sanum remedies based upon analyzing the fresh blood under dark field microscopy.

A pilot study found the reliability of blood analysis using dark field microscopy to be low and difficult to standardize.

ELECTRO-DERMAL TESTING

In the 1950s, Reinhard Voll theorized that if meridians really were energy channels, then they should be measurable. He combined acupuncture theory with a galvanometer (a device that measures differences in electrical current, also known as the galvanic skin response, which is one area of measurement in a lie detector or polygraph test) and electro-dermal testing (EDT) was born.

Also written unhyphenated (electrodermal) or as two words (electro dermal) and sometimes as *computerized electrodermal screening* (CEDS), EDT is done with a device that measures the electrical potential between two points in hope of gaining information about the animal's health. Practitioners also work on saliva and hair samples.

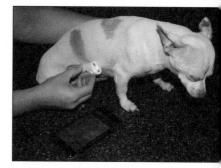

RIGHT: **Scanners use the galvanic skin response with proprietary software to approximate diagnoses and suggest remedies.**

There are numerous proprietary EDT scanning devices available. Some devices then connect via Bluetooth to a cell phone or are connected to a computer database to suggest a diagnosis and remedies. It is important to realize that the galvanic skin response depends upon the pressure the practitioner uses while scanning the patient, the quality of the skin contact with the device, and the level of moisture in the patient's skin. Different devices deployed by different practitioners on the same patient can give very different results. See *RainDrop Technique*.

Prosecutorial action has stopped EDT practice on people in some states, but marketers have repackaged their devices with new twists.

ELECTROPHORESIS

Electrophoresis is the scientific term for the movement of charged particles via an electrical field, such as one created with the application of electrodes to the skin. In conventional medicine, immunoelectrophoresis and immunochemical electrophoresis are standard tests used to assess the amount and type of immunoglobins and antibodies in the patient. In the alternative treatment setting, some practitioners assert electrophoresis assists with lymph drainage and improves the benefits of massage. Drugs or herbs are also delivered via this mechanism, similar to the manner in which dimethyl sulfoxide (DMSO) has long been used to carry substances into the body across the skin. As a transporter of supplements or other medication, electrophoresis is also referred to as *iontophoresis*.

ESOGETIC COLORPUNCTURE

German naturopath Peter Mandel developed esogetic colorpuncture, a form of acupressure using colored lights, with the treatment usually being done in conjunction with Kirlian assessment (see *Kirlian Assessment*). Although the name implies otherwise, there is no puncturing of the skin in colorpuncture, just the use of colored lights at acupuncture points, often with very little pressure as well.

HAIR ANALYSIS

Conventional research sometimes uses microscopic and chemical analysis of hair to determine the presence or absence of various chemicals, including the detection of heavy metal poisoning. In the world of alternative treatments, hair analysis is offered by practitioners who claim to be able to assess the nutritional and health status of a patient. The service is usually promoted as *hair mineral* analysis (HMA) or hair tissue mineral analysis (HTMA).

It is important not to confuse HMA with other studies of hair or fur, such as trichology (the scientific study of scalp and hair health) or DNA testing. In the latter, a hair sample is pulled to analyze the DNA in intact cells of the hair root, usually for the purpose of determining genetic traits when planning a breeding.

A veterinarian who specializes in horses asserts that 80 percent of horses either have toxic levels of heavy metals in their systems, or are deficient in minerals, or are electrolyte deficient. For about two hundred dollars, online buyers can purchase hair analysis services from this vet and mail in their animals' hair sample. Buyers receive a multipage report of the laboratory findings along with the vet's recommendations on nutritional supplementation and what he terms "detoxification." The veterinarian advertises that he need not personally see the animal. He sells special supplemental formulas that he says are created for the individual animal based on the hair analysis results, and advertises that his individually designed oral supplements can chelate heavy metals, detoxifying the horse.

One equine supplement company states hair analysis can reveal enzyme and endocrine function, inflammatory tendencies, and nutritional imbalances. Some alternative practitioners offering HMA claim to be able to assess medical problems such as allergies or stress via hair analysis. Mainstream medicine categorically advises that allergies cannot be determined through hair analysis.

Alternative practitioners for animals who tout HMA as a reliable method of screening the pet's mineral content note that fur collection is not only less invasive than having a blood sample analyzed, but that a length of hair provides a record of intakes and exposures in the past weeks and months, while blood shows only the content of the patient at the time tested.

The American Medical Association is opposed to hair analysis as a means of assessing human health. A 1985 article in the *Journal of the American Medical Association* (*JAMA*) reported that hair samples from two healthy patients sent to more than a dozen labs reaped inconsistent results, with very little agreement among the different labs on what mineral and other values were identified in the hair samples. Half the labs recommended various nutritional supplementations. The article's author, Dr. Stephen Barrett, serves as a guardian against health care fraud. He calls hair analysis a cardinal sign of quackery; one of the labs that routinely provides hair mineral analysis sued him in the summer of 2010.

In 2001, *JAMA* reported a similar experiment on HMA services, sending samples from one volunteer to multiple labs, and again the results were inconsistent, with the researchers concluding that HMA was unreliable and health care practitioners should refrain from the practice.

One medical doctor who advocates HMA decries the two studies published sixteen years apart in *JAMA* and advises that practitioners using HMA should make their lab requests to one of two labs in the United States that does not clean the hair samples. This advocate also points to a 1979 meta-analysis by the U.S., Environmental Protection Agency (EPA) that reviewed more than 400 studies using HMA from around the world.

The EPA meta-analysis concluded that if "hair and nail samples are collected, *cleaned* [emphasis added] and analyzed properly with the best analytical methods under controlled conditions by experienced personnel, the data are valid. Human hair and nails have been found to be meaningful and representative tissues for biological monitoring for most of these [antimony, arsenic, boron, cadmium, chromium, cobalt, copper, lead, mercury, nickel, selenium, tin, and vanadium] toxic metals."

Another medical doctor who recommends HMA suggests using yet a different lab and also points to the EPA meta-study as proof of the efficacy of HMA. He recommends only sending hair samples to labs that use inductively coupled plasma mass spectrometry (ICP-MS), not ICP-atomic emission spectrometry.

Mass spectrometry involves using acid to digest the hair sample, burning the now-liquefied sample, and measuring the gases given off during burning.

Analysis of hair has been used to successfully identify the presence of certain heavy metals, but the baseline or norm for many of these values is not known, making HMA for specific heavy metals a qualitative test but not a good quantitative test. There are no reference ranges for how much lead, for instance, one should expect in a horse living in a given area. There is no known appropriate value for how much zinc is acceptable in a dog's fur.

Mercury is often present in hair samples, for example, but people and animals are regularly exposed to mercury in water, food, and air. Methyl mercury can be ingested by consuming fish. A person eating several cans of tuna a day for consecutive days and weeks can develop mercury poisoning symptoms and show elevated levels of methyl mercury in tissue samples, including hair samples.

The Agency for Toxic Substances and Disease Registry (ATSDR) asserts that with the exception of methyl mercury, hair analysis testing for environmental exposure provides no insight into whether or not the tested individual has or will have health consequences from the chemical or element identified in a hair sample.

In 2002, the U.S. Centers for Disease Control and Prevention (CDC) also concluded that hair analysis was unreliable.

Hair of the Dog: Alternative Analysis

Roll over Beethoven. *Newsweek* magazine reported in 2000 that analysis of the composer's hair revealed high concentrations of lead. This finding raised speculation that lead poisoning may have caused or contributed to Ludwig van Beethoven's death. Such remarkable news helped foster interest in laboratory analysis of hair, with the alternative treatments industry—which had long been using hair analysis—promoting anew the practice of hair analysis to identify both nutritional deficiencies and the presence of toxic elements assumed to be in the body.

I borrowed a lovely dog named Maxine and completed an alternative practitioner's accompanying questionnaire, prepared to pay the fee and wait for results.

And I read a 2008 article in *Toxicology & Environmental Chemistry* which concluded that lead was not a likely contributing factor in Beethoven's illness or death. This article notes that Pb (*Pb* signifies lead in the periodic table of the elements) in hair is known to be an unreliable indicator of lead absorption because hair can be contaminated with lead externally, and further, the finding reported in *Newsweek* conflicts with the known kinetics of lead in the blood.

One alternative practitioner offering HMA for pets notes that mass spectrometry is really meant for analyzing soils. This practitioner also decries blood testing animals for diagnostic purposes (believes the practice is of little benefit to the dog) or of testing via radionics boxes (believes the practice is a poor effort to replace an experienced practitioner). This practitioner instead promotes hair analysis through dowsing, claiming to read the energy signature surrounding the fur sample and that this energy signature represents the animal's body systems.

Another alternative animal practitioner needs just one single hair from the animal and claims to then be able to remotely connect with and read the pet in perpetuity.

Some shampoos contain the same elements that are routinely tested for in HMA, such as selenium, lead, iron, or zinc. Thus, HMA services have specific guidance on how recently washed or otherwise processed sampled hair can be. They also direct people to sample from just above the nape of the neck, though this is largely a vanity issue, affording the person a well-hidden sampled area.

Animal practitioners have transferred this advice to suggesting hair be taken from an animal's lower neck. Indeed, the service I used gave specific instructions.

"Cut fur from the lower neck or breast, where she can't lick herself."

Maxine, the borrowed dog whose fur I submitted for analysis to this alternative practitioner is a fourteen-year-old female mixed breed. She's fed a premium diet and has been with the same loving family almost all of her life. Because she is aged, she gets wellness checks at her veterinarian, but she has no medical problems. She

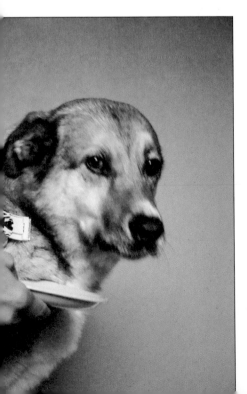

enjoys long daily walks. People would guess she's in her middle years, but they wouldn't guess she's fourteen—she acts half her age.

In completing the questionnaire on the animal's history and health complaints, I was tempted to report that Maxine suffered numerous symptoms, to see if the lab report might arrive adjusted to fit possible explanations. If I said she was lethargic, would

LEFT: **Sampling fur from the neck for hair trace mineral analysis.**

they report her low in iron? If I said that she had an assortment of nonspecific illnesses, might they claim various heavy metals were in her fur?

To be fair, a good health care provider evaluating an animal will inquire about the animal's history and its living situation, diet, and symptoms. It would be unfair of me to claim the dog had symptoms she did not in fact exhibit.

I did, however, claim I had just found her, so her diet and past exposures were completely unknown.

The HMA service I patronized claims they can analyze the presence or absence of more than half of the periodic table of elements. When I called to arrange the basic test of about two dozen minerals, the consultant immediately suggested I purchase the more expensive test of over fifty minerals.

"It's in parts per billion, whereas the basic test is only in parts per million," he said. "And of course, it tests for a lot more things, like palladium."

Palladium? Maxine, my loaner dog, could have a problem with palladium in her system?

I thought about the previous reports in *JAMA* sending samples to multiple labs. Nobody had bothered sending identical samples to the same lab. I sent two samples from Maxine to the same service, but I claimed the samples were from two different dogs. I named the second fur sample *Beethoven*.

A month later, I was still waiting for results. The service again suggested I pay for the expanded testing at a higher fee. I agreed and sent the additional funds.

Two more weeks on, the first report arrived. Beethoven was reported to be low in vanadium and high in both bismuth and iodine. Palladium was high too, although not quite in the range to place red stars on the pages of results. The measurement value of the results was listed as parts per million (ppm) equal to milligrams per kilogram (mg/kg) equal to micrograms per gram (mcg/g).

In order to detoxify Beethoven, I should change the dog's diet, including add supplements. Recommendations included avoiding iodine-rich foods like fish and kelp, adding oil to the diet, having the drinking water tested (to look for sources of contamination), increasing intake of high-protein food or adding an amino-acid nutritional supplement, and adding a basic mineral supplement and an ultra B-complex vitamin. The testing service offered dozens of supplemental products to meet these recommendations.

Finally Maxine's results arrived. While Maxine's results also showed high in bismuth and iodine, she did not show low in vanadium or high in palladium. Also, many of the elements in Maxine's results that were listed within the lab's listed normal range were significantly different from the Beethoven sample.

Element	Laboratory's Acceptable Range	Maxine's Result	Beethoven's Result
ppm=mg/kg=mcg/g			
calcium	400–2,200	1279.74	944.45
magnesium	87–321	148.56	117.42
chromium	0.01–0.85	0.09	0.04
cobalt	< 0.35	0.04	0.02
copper	11–70	19.22	28.94
iodine	0.24–1.99	3.9	3.25
iron	6–72	13.47	10.71
vanadium	0.01–0.4	0.02	0.01
strontium	0.35–6	2.95	1.63
aluminum	< 66	3.74	2.59
bismuth	< 0.03	0.46	0.49
palladium	< 0.04	0.01	0.04

The nutritional and detoxification recommendations were similar for Maxine and Beethoven, and the results were not startlingly different, but they were different enough to raise my eyebrows. The fur samples were collected from the same location on the same dog on the same day. Shouldn't her calcium and copper levels, for example, have been the same?

Were I truly concerned about an animal's body chemistry, I would seek blood testing.

HELIOTHERAPY

Also called *phototherapy*, heliotherapy is the use of lights to treat an animal. It has some crossover with color therapy, as many practitioners are very specific about what color of light they choose to treat a particular complaint. Ayurvedic crossover comes in when practitioners employ colors that they correlate to specific chakras.

LED (light-emitting diode) devices are used by some practitioners who claim they have fewer side effects than do lasers. The scattered beam of LEDs, also called a noncoherent source (as opposed to the focused coherent beam of a laser), does not penetrate tissue as deeply as does a laser. In addition to use on behavioral complaints, they are promoted for physical concerns such as wound healing.

HYDROTHERAPY

Literally meaning treatment with water, hydrotherapy can also refer to medicated wet soaks or packs (such as castor oil, Epsom salt, or plain water) applied to an area of the body. Classical naturopathy strongly embraced hydrotherapy. It is often done by nearly complete immersion in water but may be in combination with physical therapy, such as massage in general or watsu in specific, or with physical exercise, such as swimming a sore or injured dog.

This type of rehabilitative exercise hydrotherapy may also be called *aquatic therapy*.

A dog who is unsure about swimming will likely benefit from going with a dog who is a happy swimmer. While accessing a man-made equine hydrotherapy facility is expensive, horses have been given hydrotherapy with great success.

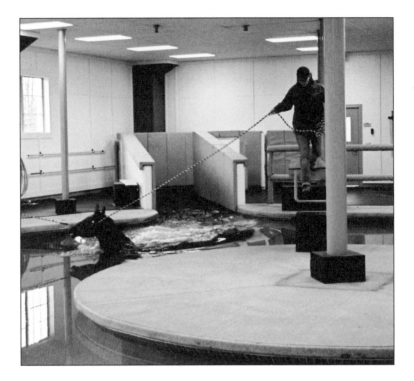

ABOVE: **Hydrotherapy. Some treatments classified as alternatives are also considered conventional mainstream therapies.**

Any animal who is asked to immerse should be carefully monitored for safety, as the swimming area must not have dangerous debris concealed underwater on which the animal could accidentally strike his legs. Also, the animal must have an immediate safe exit from the area.

Something that feels good to us can be extremely uncomfortable to an animal. Be warned that hot tubs warm enough to be pleasant soaking for a human (perhaps 103° F) are inherently dangerous to dogs, who can easily get hyperthermic.

HYPERBARIC OXYGEN TREATMENT

Hyperbaric oxygen treatment (HBOT) involves placing the patient in a chamber that is pressurized with pure oxygen. It can be effective in treating anaerobic bacterial infections. It is an approved therapy for people suffering from gangrene, cerebral abscess, air embolism, inadequately oxygenated tissue, or decompression sickness. The latter occurs only to those who have suffered sudden, extreme decompression, which is achievable only through rising too fast from either deep-sea diving or a very deep mine tunnel, or from being in a jet at high altitude with cabin pressure failure. Obviously, only the latter could apply to an animal as a means of developing decompression sickness. In humans, HBOT is used as an alternative treatment for everything from AIDS to autism, although there is no proof it definitively helps any condition for which it is not approved. Similarly, HBOT is sometimes administered to animals for problems that are not known to be treatable through hyperbaric oxygen.

BELOW: **Hyperbaric chambers large enough to accommodate a horse are becoming more common.**

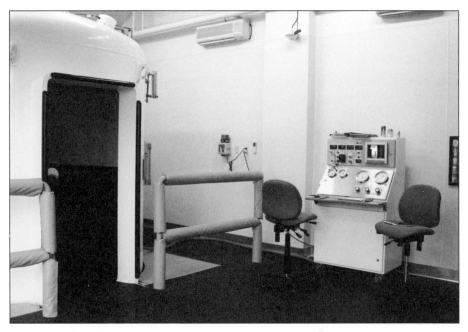

There are facilities with hyperbaric chambers large enough to accommodate a horse. The horse will be well groomed, as any oil (from previous grooming products) could present a fire hazard under the pressurized oxygen environment. While oxygen is not flammable, it dramatically increases the burn rate of what would normally be an incidental spark or heat of no real concern, such as static electricity or friction from rubbing. For this reason, an animal is often hosed down to increase humidity in the air near him, thus reducing the chance of static electricity, and a shod horse would have his shoes covered in tape so they could not strike together and create a spark. Also, the animal would not wear a leather collar or halter, but a clean cotton one, as leather often retains old oil products. The treatment could last thirty minutes to two hours, and an animal may receive five, ten, or twenty treatments.

HBOT complications include oxygen toxicity seizures.

INFRASOUND

Infrasound (low-frequency waves) is used in applications similar to that of ultrasound techniques, both diagnostically and therapeutically. As the machine generates sound waves and outputs the infrasound through a wand applied directly to the patient's skin, an image is formed by the infrasound machine on a monitor.

Unlike ultrasound, infrasound does not tend to generate heat. Promoters recommend the device as a treatment for almost any condition and sell it to untrained personnel. While infrared thermography (the use of an infrared device to display temperature changes in the tissues) has shown temperature changes post infrasound therapy sessions, there is no concrete research demonstrating efficacy in such broad applications as the promoters suggest.

Infratonic therapy is a synonym for infrasound treatment.

INTRINSIC DATA FIELD ANALYSIS

These electronic machines are intended to analyze data from the patient regarding numerous body functions. At the same time, they are sold with warnings that they are not to be used to diagnose, assess, or otherwise substitute for competent medical care. This is due to the legal ramifications of making unsubstantiated claims. Some practitioners equate the intrinsic data field concept to an aura or electromagnetic field. There are numerous such devices for sale and employed by various practitioners of alternative treatments for animals.

IRIDOLOGY

Formerly called iridodiagnosis, iridology is the belief that the body can be mapped on the iris (the colored part of the eye), so that the source of a problem can be identified. It is essentially palm reading done on the eye, with health instead of fortune being the topic of discussion. The theory may stem from marks in the iris (the iris can freckle like skin does) being correlated to a bodily complaint. While some iridologists insist that iridology is not intended to be diagnostic, the purpose of iridology is clearly not to be therapeutic in the sense of delivering treatment, but instead it is a means to assess the body.

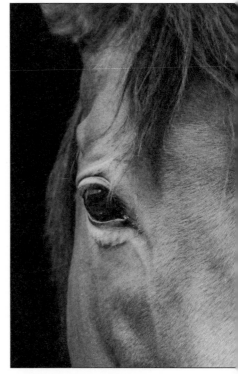

ABOVE: **Iridology. Can the body be assessed by studying the iris (colored part of the eye)?**

KINESIOLOGY

Kinesiology, the study of movement, was, and continues to be, an established field of scientific inquiry sometimes called academic kinesiology. Chiropractor George Goodheart originated what he termed *applied kinesiology* in the 1960s. The similarity

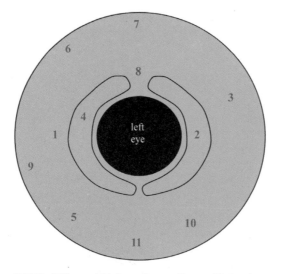

1-circulatory system
2-digestive system
3-endocrine system
4-excretory system
5-hepatic function
6-lymphatic system
7-mental function
8-nervous system
9-pulmonary function
10-renal function
11-reproductive system

ABOVE: **Different iridology charts offer conflicting interpretations.**

in the terms *academic* and *applied kinesiology* results in confusion of the two dissimilar fields. Goodheart's applied kinesiology consisted of manual muscle testing that sought to find a dysfunctional muscle and manipulate the muscle to restore normal function. Some kinesiologists choose a supplement, treatment, or food for animal patients by having the owner hold out an arm while touching the animal, then the practitioner pushes on the owner's arm in an attempt to ascertain the animal's resistance to, or acceptance of, a suggested treatment. This is also called surrogate muscle response testing.

Other practitioners attempt to to do kinesiology on the animal by writing, for example, various dietary suggestions on index cards then placing the cards on the animal and trying to determine the animal's reaction to the suggestions.

Although the practice is not scientifically grounded, numerous animal chiropractors, naturopaths, homeopaths, and specialists advertise their use of kinesiology and report good results.

Kinergetics is a combination form of kinesiology and mystical energy healing practiced in about a dozen of the United States as well as in Australia, Singapore, Switzerland, South Africa, Norway,

Spain, China, Canada, England, Israel, Hong Kong, Netherlands, Malaysia, Brazil, and Germany. It has been extended to animal care and includes muscle response testing. Practitioners believe they can successfully treat allergies, anxiety, and many other physical and mental problems.

KIRLIAN ASSESSMENT

In 1939, Russian inventor Seymon Davidovich Kirlian and his wife Valentina Khrisonovna Kirliana rediscovered that a subject on a photographic plate exposed to voltage left an image on the plate. The physics behind this is due to the corona effect—with corona here being a halo shape. A corona discharge is an electrical discharge accompanied by ionization of the immediate atmosphere. This is the underlying principle of xerography (modern photocopying).

Corona effect occurs in nature in addition to being man-made. In meteorological terms, Saint Elmo's fire is an example of coronal discharge occurring during lightning (an electrical storm) at the ends of pointed objects such as a ship's mast, when charged or ionized plasma appears to be flame, often blue in color.

The images or auras seen in Kirlian photograms (*photogram* is a more proper term than *photograph*, as the image is an outline, not a photo) are luminous radiations outlining the body or body part examined. By the late 1950s, supernatural or metaphysical connotations were applied to Kirlian photographs, with practitioners attempting to assess the well-being of a subject by studying the image produced. Some modern alternative veterinarians and other practitioners use Kirlian assessment, for example taking an image of a dog's paw before and after treatment with therapy such as crystals or chakra alignment, to demonstrate efficacy. Some practitioners term the practice *energy emission analysis* (EEA), but the name *Kirlian* is more commonly encountered.

Kirlian photography or assessment is often confused with *aural photography* although the two are different processes (see *Aural Photography* under *Mystical*).

LARVAL THERAPY

Larval therapy is also known as maggot therapy, though it would more accurately be termed maggot debridement or wound debridement using maggots. To debride a wound is to remove infected and necrotic (dead) tissue, or by-products of infection such as pus, in order to enable the wound to heal. Fly larvae, also known as maggots, are the small worm-like stage of flies that emerge from fly eggs. The larvae feed on infected and necrosing tissue.

Debriding a wound via applying live maggots to the wound is an ancient practice that was employed on multiple continents. Through the 1800s in the Western world, it was not uncommon that maggots found on wounds were allowed to remain to do their natural work, or maggots were introduced to wounds in order to promote healing.

It is important to note that unlike the broad spectrum of alternative treatments that are classified as alternatives because there is insufficient scientific data to demonstrate that they work, the medical application of maggots to debride a wound does work. The larvae literally eat up the infection in a wound, then migrate out, perhaps leaving behind unidentified constituents that also aid in healing.

Numerous developments led to maggots losing their hospital job. Medical science moved out of its infancy. Germ theory was recognized. The importance of aseptic technique was accepted, and antibiotics were discovered. Finally, there is the ick factor of using live bugs on a live patient who is already suffering with an awful wound.

In modern times, in a very few medical facilities, sterilized larvae of the common green bottle fly (*Phaeniciasericata*, also known by its older Latin name, *Luciliasericata*) are carefully introduced into a moist wound and bandaged to prevent drying out or escape of the larvae. The maggots are purchased from a medical vendor that has sterilized the larvae to ensure that they are not carrying disease or germs which they could then introduce into the wound.

Maggots have the ability to enter, for example, an abscessed hoof, and clean out the infection while leaving the healthy tissue undisturbed. At Rood and Riddle, the esteemed veterinary hospital in

Lexington, Kentucky, Dr. Scott Morrison has patients that benefit from maggots every week. Practitioners sometimes soak the affected area with chlorine dioxide to better enable the maggots to take to the wound.

If an alternative practitioner offered to introduce into a wound a batch of maggots that had not been medically sterilized, the animal patient would be at significant risk for a host of disease and secondary infection. Myiasis, the infestation of *live* tissue with larvae, is one risk of maggot therapy. For these reasons, maggot debridement (also known as larval therapy or maggot therapy), should only be sought from an established veterinarian who uses medical grade maggots.

LASER THERAPY

Also called *LLLT* (low-level laser therapy) and *cold laser*, medical laser units have been around long enough to have a number of testimonials about their efficacy, while they still lack scientifically demonstrated results. They are used in acupuncture (actually a form of acupressure when done with a laser) and in treating scar tissue or general wounds in an effort to promote circulation and healing.

Cold lasers are not the high-powered lasers used for surgery, but rather are low-powered versions that do not burn the skin, although they can still burn sensitive tissue, such as the eye.

Veterinary laser devices, selling for over six hundred dollars, are marketed freely to untrained personnel thus laser therapy sessions may be offered by various practitioners. See also *Neural Therapy*.

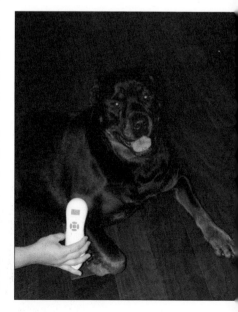

RIGHT: In treatment, the laser would be directly on the animal, thus the red light would be less visible; the cold laser is slightly angled here for demonstration purposes.

MAGNETIC THERAPY

Magnets are applied in blankets, special wraps, or individually to an injured area. The practice of using these static magnets, which are just like the magnets one puts on a refrigerator to hold a note, and are biologically inert, (as opposed to dynamic magnets focused on specific frequencies to perform transcranial magnetic stimulation in a specific hospital setting) is old and remains unproven for chronic complaints. Proponents believe the magnets stimulate circulation, thus promoting healing. Others believe that magnetic polarity influences the naturally electrically charged chemicals in the body.

The U.S. National Institutes of Health reports magnet strength is measured in gauss (G) or tesla units, with one tesla equal to 10,000 G. For comparison, commercial magnets marketed for pain relief are usually 300–5,000 G, which is much stronger than the Earth's magnetic field and much weaker than an MRI (magnetic resonance imaging). The NIH noted one 2007 study that did show a positive correlation between the immediate use of very strong magnets on an acute injury and the reduction of swelling in the injury, yet in a study of people complaining of foot pain, all were given an insert to wear in their shoes, with half of the subjects given a magnetic insert and half given an insert without the magnets—more than half of the test subjects reported improvement in their foot pain, but there was no difference between the group who were given the magnetic insert and those given the placebo.

Pulsed (also called *pulsating*) *electromagnetic field* (*PEMF*) is a variation of magnetic therapy in which the magnets are powered through

BELOW: **A pulsed electromagnetic field (PEMF) is generated by a specialized device which can be purchased by anyone.**

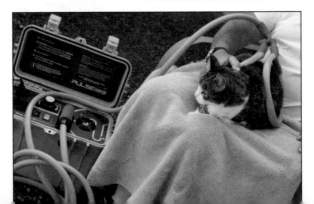

an electrical current in the hope of improved benefit. PEMF may be administered in a large device resembling a pipe, in which the animal rests while a generator produces the pulsing electromagnetic field, or the device may be a mat large enough and strong enough to permit a horse to stand on it. There is usually no perceptible feeling for the patient even though a verifiable PEMF is present. It is touted as a physical therapy, a vibrational therapy, a method to increase oxygen flow and stimulate healing, and a method to reestablish the proper cellular electric potential.

MESOTHERAPY

Michel Pistor, a French physician, began mesotherapy in the 1950s, inserting very small needles into the mesoderm (middle layer of skin) of human patients in an effort to transfer minute amounts of saline, lidocaine, homeopathic remedies, or other substances directly under the skin, in the area targeted for treatment. The treatment was later touted as a cure for cellulite and is sometimes used without attempting to pass any medicine or supplement through or on the needle into the skin—essentially a form of deep acupuncture.

Mesotherapy is most commonly given to animals as an adjunct for treating pain or muscle spasms, in an effort to interrupt the pain cycle thus providing relief.

MICROAMPERAGE/MICROCURRENT ELECTRICAL NEUROMUSCULAR STIMULATION (MENS)

A microamp is one millionth of an amp. Although generating a smaller stimulation, MENS units are used in the same applications as TENS units, but most especially advocated for wound healing. Alpha-Stim is one proprietary form of MENS/TENS.

MOXIBUSTION

Moxibustion is the burning of mugwort, an herb, on or near a patient in hope of a therapeutic benefit. The practice has been credited by believers as a panacea, able to help with everything from dreams to cleansing the blood to redirecting a fetus that is improperly positioned. Mugwort belongs to the genus Artemisia, with many varieties found in Eurasia and the Americas.

The herb may be loose or rolled into a cigar for burning. Some practitioners intentionally burn and scar the patient while others burn the mugwort on a thin slice of ginger to prevent burning the patient. The practitioner may try to warm or stimulate acupuncture points through moxibustion or may not actually even touch the burning herb to the animal.

Moxibustion has been extended by some practitioners to herbs other than mugwort.

MUSCLE RESPONSE TESTING

Muscle response testing attempts to determine weakness or imbalance and thereby diagnose a health problem and decide upon a course of treatment. One example is a practitioner pushing on a patient's limbs and assessing the patient's muscular resistance. Practitioners who perform muscle response testing on animals often use a human surrogate who is touching the animal at the same time the practitioner tests the human surrogate, as they believe the animal's muscle responses can be assessed through the human surrogate. Practitioners may attempt to do response testing by placing note cards on the animal and attempting to discern the animal's acceptance or rejection of, for example, a supplement, by doing muscle response testing after placing the written suggestion on the animal. See the section on *Kinesiology*.

NAMBUDRIPAD ALLERGY ELIMINATION TECHNIQUE (NAET)

Devi Nambudripad is a registered nurse and chiropractor who reports she discovered and developed a treatment system for human allergy sufferers involving around twenty treatment sessions of mild exposure to an allergen at the same time acupuncture is performed. After each treatment session, the patient must avoid the allergen for twenty-five hours. In the late 1990s, the NAET was adapted by Roger and Rahmie Valentine for treatment on animals. They expanded the medical term *allergy* to include what they term *emotional allergies*, and claim success with their treatment. They also give three-day seminars that certify practitioners in the technique, including an understanding of TCM, kinesiology, muscle response testing, and more.

NATUROPATHY

Naturopathy is a whole medical system that was largely cast aside when rapid advances in modern medicine were achieved, but it is having a resurgence in the last few decades. It generally seeks to avoid conventional pharmaceuticals and surgery, advocating natural cure instead. See the therapists section—*What Is a Naturopath?*—for more information on naturopathy.

NEURAL THERAPY

German medical doctors and brothers Walter and Ferdinand Huneke devised neural therapy in the 1920s after Ferdinand injected their sister with a small amount of procaine (a local anesthetic) subcutaneously, creating a weal in anticipation of doing a larger injection. See *Aquapuncture: Weal of Fortune* for further explanation on therapeutic weals.

Ms. Huneke's migraine stopped after the small procaine injection. With this, neural therapy, also called *segmental therapy*, was born. It is advocated for recalcitrant pain complaints, although some alternative veterinarians promote the treatment for other complaints, even for allergies. Proponents believe neural therapy reenergizes or repolarizes nerve cells that are disturbed, hyperreactive, or essentially short-circuiting. They call the problem area an *interference zone*. Some practitioners suggest needleless neural therapy via lasers.

NEWCASTLE TREATMENT

Canine distemper is a highly contagious, often-fatal virus that affects dogs with poor immunity. There is an effective vaccine for the disease. Retired veterinarian Alson Sears claims to have cured canine distemper through off-label use of the Newcastle disease vaccine.

Newcastle disease is a virus with a high mortality rate that affects birds with flu-like symptoms. Newcastle disease was discovered in the 1920s, and it has several strains. It does not seem to transfer outside of avians, but epidemics sweep through chicken populations, for example, affecting food supply to chicken consumers. There is no treatment for the disease, but an effective vaccine was developed.

Sears's Newcastle treatment for canine distemper involves creating a serum by injecting a healthy dog with the bird vaccine, then taking serum from the healthy dog and injecting it into the dog with canine distemper. Some supporters of the treatment call it Serum X. A variant of the Newcastle treatment involves using the bird vaccine directly on the distemper-affected dog.

The Newcastle treatment has never been evaluated in a controlled clinical environment through standard, double-blind testing, and there is very little support or recognition for this treatment in mainstream veterinary medicine. The Newcastle disease virus (NDV) itself—not the vaccine—has been shown to have some oncolytic (cancer-killing) ability and is being actively studied as a cancer-fighting agent.

It is worth noting that dogs with canine distemper who receive excellent veterinary care are given supportive or palliative care: dogs that had been in a contaminated environment are cleaned up, dehydrated dogs get fluids, dogs with secondary bacterial pneumonia get antibiotics. Supportive care is standard with viral infections, as viruses are not cured directly; the body must defeat the virus. Distemper dogs who have received the Newcastle treatment are likewise getting attentive supportive care, which is one reason why the Newcastle treatment cannot be known to be effective until it is actually tested.

NUTRIGENOMICS

Nutrigenomics is a portmanteau of *nutrition* and *genomics*; genomics refers to the study of genomes. A genome is the complete

DNA or cellular code of an organism. It is known that while an animal may have a gene for a particular malady or disease, the gene may not be expressed (activated). The field of modifying which genes are expressed is called epigenetics. The idea behind nutrigenomics (also called nutriepigenomics), is that individual animals differ in their nutritional needs and their responses to different diets, and because dietary factors affect which genes are expressed, tailoring a diet very specifically to the individual animal is key to achieving good health.

Nutrigenomics is an emerging scientific field that has been co-opted in the realm of alternative treatments, with a number of unproven claims and recommendations. At least one major purveyor of nutrigenomics asserts that chicken is unhealthy for dogs. Many also assert that animals should only be fed organic food, should never be given genetically modified food, and other overbroad claims, such as wheat, soy, or corn is bad for all animals. While it is true that certain Irish setters are gluten intolerant, it is not true that in general wheat is bad for all animals.

One alternative nutrigenomics method to determine an individual diet is through testing the saliva (see *Saliva Testing*) in the hope of discerning dietary sensitivities. While laboratory testing of mammal saliva is a scientifically confirmed practice to identify, for example, blood type, there is little scientific evidence to back the claim that most dietary sensitivities are detectable in the saliva. Overall, research in cutting-edge science, such as nutrigenomics, lags in veterinary medicine. There are tremendous gaps in the field and a lot of guesswork in trying to fill in those gaps, making it challenging for animal owners to discern what is known and what is opinion or mere guessing. Readers are cautioned not to be misled by bad science.

In the United States, relatively few home genetic swab (saliva) tests have FDA approval. Numerous kits available for purchase to supposedly enable nutrigenomics counseling are not FDA approved because a genetic test is considered to be a medical device only if it is a freestanding kit sold to a laboratory, whereas many labs make up their own kits, so the latter are not regulated and have not had to prove their efficacy.

The US Government Accounting Office bought multiple at-home test packages (ranging from under one hundred dollars to more than a thousand dollars) from several different vendors that offer saliva testing and provide what the vendors claim to be tailored nutrigenomics counseling based on the results of the saliva test. The GAO took multiple saliva samples from an adult and a baby, then sent the samples in as though they were actually from twelve different individuals. The nine samples that actually all came from the same person resulted in variable nutritional recommendations. One vendor offered expensive supplements to repair what it claimed was the patient's damaged DNA.

It is clear that the nutrigenomics vendors made recommendations based on the consumer-completed questionnaire, rather than the saliva sample in some areas. On a profile that the GAO listed as belonging to a smoker, the nutrigenomics service recommended the patient stop smoking; on the sample that was claimed to be from a nonsmoker, the nutrigenomics report suggested the person continue to not smoke. Testing the alternative practitioners that offer these services to our pets is likely to yield similar results.

While it is emphasized that nutrigenomics is a legitimate, emerging field of science and there is tremendous value in a healthy diet, the current state of direct-to-consumer alternative nutrigenomics is fraught with dubious claims.

OZONE THERAPY

Not to be confused with *zone therapy*, ozone therapy is, strictly speaking, the administration of extra oxygen created by an ozone (O_3) generator.

Some practitioners use hydrogen peroxide, (H_2O_2), as a means of adding oxygen to the tissues and may term this treatment ozone therapy as well. Note that medical/food-grade hydrogen peroxide may be used, which is a 35-percent-strength solution while the peroxide most people have in their homes, purchased at a typical grocery store, is 3 percent. Also, remember that simple household peroxide works as an emetic in most patients.

Neither O_3 nor H_2O_2 should be confused with oxygen, the medical gas used to treat hypoxic patients, which is often referred to as O_2. Oxygen therapy may also be administered in a hyperbaric chamber. Neither oxygen administration nor hyperbaric oxygen treatment (HBOT) are necessarily alternative treatments, but rather, these are conventional treatments (although HBOT is relatively uncommon) that are sometimes used in an alternative manner, for problems not recognized by mainstream medicine as treatable by oxygen. Ozone and peroxide *are* alternative treatments.

Both oral and intravenous administration methods of ozone and hydrogen peroxide are used, with the intravenous method being more common, more invasive, and more dangerous. Practitioners use ozone therapy when they think the tissues need extra oxygen, such as in the treatment of some cancers and severe viruses. Proponents say the pathogen might be unable to survive in the presence of the added oxygen. It is certainly true that ozone and peroxide are reactive. They kill many biologics in vitro, but in vivo—within the body—the effects are not controlled. Ozone therapy is a disproved alternative cancer treatment for people but remains one of the modalities recognized by the American Holistic Veterinary Medical Association.

PHOTONIC THERAPY

Australian veterinarian Brian McLaren developed an instrument for performing acupuncture with a red, non-laser light. Acupoint treatment with various devices is increasingly common throughout the world, but McLaren's photonic therapy is most common in Australia. As such, photonic therapy is more specific than phototherapy, which simply refers to alternative treatment done with lights, including red lights.

In the United States, the treatment is known as *low energy photon therapy (LEPT)*, and it is administered through lasers or LEDs for a wide variety of animal problems. Owner-perceived improvement in a pet receiving LEPT is likely due to caregiver-placebo response, or the nonspecific effects of the treatment, such as a calm soothing therapy room with kind handling.

PROLOTHERAPY

Prolotherapy, also called *sclerotherapy*, is similar to mesotherapy, although the targeted area for injection is usually deeper and usually supporting tissues of a joint, such as a ligament. The name stands for proliferative therapy and is hoped to help proliferate or reconstruct tissue. A sclerosant (injected irritant) of sugar or saline solution, vitamins, herbal preparation is injected into the treatment area, stimulating an inflammatory response, which is hoped to enhance healing. Animals have certainly been subjected to a lot of injections that are hoped to benefit them, but science-based medicine does not support these injections.

QXCI QUANTUM HEALING

The Holistic Animal Therapy Association of Australia is perhaps the only organization centered on animal care to recognize QXCI quantum healing. The initials naming the device stand for Quantum Xrroid Consciousness Interface. It is promoted as an expanded bio-feedback machine intended to analyze essentially every bodily function in an effort to create wellness. Vendors recommend it for pets as well as people, but the unapproved device is uncommon.

While biofeedback, a human therapy intended to enhance relaxation, is sometimes supported with machines that give supporting data (such as pulse) or changes in skin resistance, when these machines are intended to diagnose or treat an ailment for which they cannot be shown to plausibly diagnose or treat, they can be illegal in the United States.

RADIONICS

Albert Abrams, an entrepreneur of the late 1800s, developed the concept that would become radionics. Like *intrinsic data field analysis* units, radionics machines are devices that are meant to detect harmonics and vibrations radiating from the body, and analyze the data received in order to offer a diagnosis and prognosis. In some cases, the radionics device is claimed to then treat the patient electronically.

While some radionics promoters suggest the devices as an adjunct to conventional care, others claim it as a suppressed-by-the-majority wonder that can cure all. Some radionics-type devices are referred to as Rife machines, for Royal Raymond Rife, an inventor.

The Radionic Association of the United Kingdom notes that radionic healers use extrasensory perception (ESP) in addition to a radionics device in their work.

RAINDROP TECHNIQUE

Raindrop Technique (also written as rainDrop) is a trademarked therapy developed by D. Gary Young, who founded Young Living Essential Oils, a multilevel-marketing company that offers trademarked essential oils (see *Essential Oils*), and a training program for its practitioners. Young claimed to have developed his method in the 1980s after working with a Lakota medicine man named Wallace Black Elk. Young's method builds on the beliefs promoted in Vita Flex (see *Vita Flex*, which the YLEO company restyled as *vitaflex*), and centers on the use of essential oils in topical application. Raindrop technique is generally intended to promote healing.

Young (deceased) received an online degree in naturopathy from the now defunct Bernadine University, as well as a master's in nutrition. He was charged criminally with practicing medicine without a license. His company has received multiple warnings from the FDA after practitioners and promotional materials asserted the oils could, among other things, treat Ebola, prevent cancer, and protect against tetanus. The company was fined for violating the Endangered Species

Act after it imported rosewood oil that had been harvested from protected Brazilian rosewood trees (*Aniba roseaodora*) from Peru.

The Young Living Essential Oils company sells hundreds of different blended and unblended oils, in addition to diffusers and other products to use with its essential oils, plus publications, DVDs, and training courses. Currently, the training program is overseen by the YLEO company's Center for Aromatherapy Research and Education (CARE, Inc.). One part of the training program to become a certified CARE instructor is a 160-question take-home test that the student has two years to complete.

Practitioners may also scan patients with a galvanic skin response (GSR, see *electrodermal testing*) device that works with the practitioner's cellular phone to suggest remedies. The combination of such a specific regimen of how to apply proprietary oils, perhaps after using the proprietary GSR device that approaches a diagnostic system, places raindrop technique in the *Other* category. Although originally developed for application on people, the raindrop technique was readily transferred to animals, and some practitioners now base their business on animal care with the raindrop technique.

A raindrop technique session takes about one hour. Practitioners usually work with an array of oils, including two proprietary blends (called Aroma Siez and Valor), plus seven unblended oils: basil (*Ocimum basilicum*), cypress (*Cupressus sempervirens*), marjoram (*Origanum majorana*), peppermint (*Mentha piperita*), thyme (*Thymus vulgaris*), oregano (*Origanum compactum*), and wintergreen (*Gaultheria procumbens*).

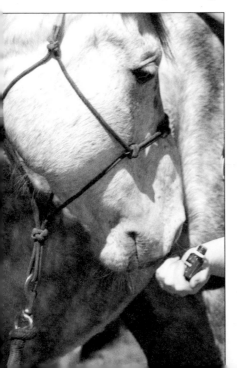

LEFT: **In raindrop technique, the therapist presents each essential oil to the animal as an offer before it is applied.**

Prior to applying an oil, raindrop technique practitioners offer each remedy by showing it to the animal. Application of the oil is done by dropping it onto the animal's body from several inches above, so that the oil falls like a raindrop onto the skin. Unlike most other essential oil practitioners, in raindrop technique, undiluted oils are applied directly to skin. If the animal's skin then exhibits a raised weal or other skin reaction that would be viewed by veterinarians as evidence of irritation, the practitioners assert that it is instead evidence of toxins being released from the body.

The raindrop technique teaches practitioners to rub circles in their own palms a specific number of times and in specific directions, and then to do so on the patient. Some practitioners assert the reason for this is to excite the molecules in the oil in hope of making the patient less susceptible to disease. Other practitioners incorporate spiritual or religious elements into the procedures.

Some patients, such as the very young, the elderly, and thin-skinned individuals, are more likely to have an adverse reaction to essential oils, especially undiluted oils used directly on the skin. Also, it is possible that some essential oils are endocrine disruptors or otherwise toxic.

There are no double-blind, randomized, peer-reviewed, large-sample studies that support the asserted theorized benefits of raindrop technique.

BELOW: **A drop of essential oil is allowed to fall onto the animal like a raindrop before being worked into the skin.**

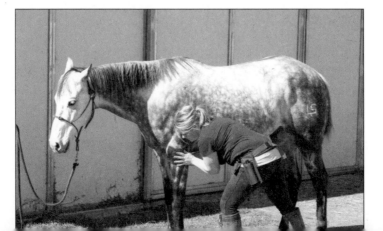

REBA TESTING

ReBa testing is the use of a device developed by medical doctor and naturopath Reimar Banis to test a patient for energy blockages that might contribute to illnesses. The device is attached to an extremity via an electrode and is purported to measure brain wave frequencies, which proponents believe correlate to four energy levels they identify as the vital, emotional, mental, and causal levels.

Also called *psychosomatic energetics* or *polyfrequency spectrum testing*, ReBa testing is promoted among some animal practitioners as a means to select the best homeopathic remedy for the pet. See *What is a Homeopath?* to fully understand homeopathic remedies and how they are made.

One practitioner calls the levels revealed by ReBa testing *chakras* and notes an example of results to be that an animal showing chakra seven might mean that the animal has epilepsy or an eye problem or an ear problem.

SALIVA TESTING

Saliva testing is the practice of examining a sample of an animal's saliva in an effort to assess dietary sensitivities or other information about the animal's health. It is strongly promoted in alternative applications of nutrigenomics (see *Nutrigenomics*). As the mouth is the beginning of the gastrointestinal tract, it is reasoned that there, in the saliva, we could scan for antibodies, thus identifying sensitivity or intolerance to specific foods that would then be avoided.

A veterinary dermatologist tested the saliva testing service by submitting a dozen individual samples: one sample was tap water, some samples were saliva from dogs with known allergies or sensitivities, and some samples were saliva from dogs with no dietary difficulties. The saliva testing service reported that all twelve samples showed animals with dietary sensitivities to beef, corn, milk, and wheat. While the field of saliva testing may improve, at this time it is unreliable.

The best standard in medicine for determining food sensitivities is careful dietary testing. The animal is placed on an elimination diet for a set time period, then other foods are reintroduced one at a time over an isolated period of time to determine which food is causing the animal problems.

SANUM REMEDIES

Günther Enderlein, born 1872, was an entomologist who posited the theory of pleomorphism, that microorganisms such as bacterium and fungi could change their shape into another form. His theory split early microbiology, with one school of thought following Enderlein and one following Louis Pasteur and others. Pasteur and company turned out to be correct; individual bacteria are monomorphic (of one shape) and do not dramatically change shape and exist in numerous morphologies or forms.

In modern times, pleomorphism is understood to mean *varying* size or shape, but not a *change* or *morphing* of shape. However, some alternative practitioners still advance Enderlein's theory of pleomorphism.

Extending oral homeopathy to injections, Enderlein diluted microbes at homeopathic proportions and then injected his mixtures into patients. See *What is a Homeopath?* to fully understand homeopathic remedies and how they are made. Enderlein founded a company called Sanum (from the Latin *sanus*, meaning "health") to promote his homeopathic remedies originally distilled from biologicals. Sanum remedies are still offered by alternative animal health practitioners in the U.K. and Continental Europe. In Canada, *polysan* remedies (a mix of several Sanum remedies) are offered by some alternative pet care practitioners. Those practitioners may choose a Sanum remedy or polysan via dark field microscopy.

SCENAR

Self-controlled energy-neuro-adaptive regulators (SCENAR), are handheld devices developed in Russia by Alexander Karasev between the 1970s and 1990s. A Scenar device is essentially a MENS or TENS unit purported to stimulate the brain and healing processes with electronic signals. Proponents see the device as different from other devices that impart electrical stimulation in that they view the Scenar as creating a feedback between the body and brain—biofeedback— instead of merely placing impulses on the skin.

Modifications to Scenar-type devices have resulted in products known generically and by trade names such as COSMODIC, DiaDENS, zooDENS, or other variations of the initials involved in various acronyms of the devices. The name Scenar is used to generally refer to both the therapy and the device.

Proponents find the devices to be useful for treating almost any complaint of illness or injury. The FDA has not approved Scenar or Scenar-type devices as a treatment or diagnostic device, so they are sold in the United States to the general public as biofeedback machines, with practitioners skirting legality issues even as they expand the use of Scenars and offer treatment services as Scenar administrators.

SONIC THERAPY

Many people use sonic therapy in the form of playing music to soothe or settle an animal. Many stables keep a radio on in the barn in the belief that it calms the horses. It is reported that cows may release more milk when pleasant music is played. As an alternative treatment, sonic therapy may be extended to those who use tuning forks in acupressure or massage treatment. Not to be confused with *sonography*.

STEM CELL THERAPY

Stem cells are cells in living beings that can self-renew and differentiate into other types of cells. Stem cell therapy, also called cell therapy or regenerative medicine, involves taking stem cells from another animal (called an allogeneic donation) or from the patient (termed an autologous donation); the stem cells are concentrated through procedures in a laboratory, then injected into the patient in hopes of alleviating an injury or disease. Some clinics may also take a blood donation from the patient, spin the blood sample down to a platelet-rich plasma (PRP) and mix the isolated stem cells with the platelet-rich plasma.

Many people have the vague notion that all stem cells can become any type of cell, thus could be used to fix almost any problem. Degenerating joint? Inject stem cells so that the dog can rebuild his own knee, the cat can rebuild its arthritic spine. It sounds wonderful and there is significant promising research in the area of stem cells, however, there are numerous stem cell therapies offered that must be classified as alternative treatments because they are fundamentally unproven or, worse, known to be ineffective. Human patients have been blinded by unproven stem cell therapies. In other cases, arrests have been made for fraud.

The truth is, there are different kinds of stem cells. A hematopoietic (blood-forming) stem cell in living bone marrow creates different kinds of blood cells, while a neural stem cell in the brain naturally creates brain cells. True, manipulations in a laboratory setting have enabled embryonic stem cells to become other types of cells, but these pluripotent and induced pluripotent cells also have a record of growing without control, thus sparking tumors.

Stem cells in an adult are tissue-specific—they cannot necessarily become any type of cell, and they change somewhat throughout an individual's life. Your old dog is not making the same stem cells he did as a youngster. These stem cells are multipotent, like the aforementioned stem cells in the bone marrow that can make platelets or white blood cells or red blood cells, but they are not able to make any type of cell in the body (pluripotent).

Stromal cells are cells that can be taken from the stroma (connective tissue surrounding organs) or fat. They are also called mesenchymal stromal cells or mesenchymal stem cells, and both terms are abbreviated as MSCs. Stromal cells have been made to grow into other types of cells in a laboratory, thus show some stem cell characteristics, but are not yet fully understood and have not at this point been proved beneficial in treatment. A study of horses with injured tendons who received embryonic stem cells and MSCs showed that the embryonic stem cells migrated throughout the injury while the MSCs did not, and that ten days after injection, less than 5 percent of the MSCs survived.

Stem cell therapy is not benign, it is invasive. Note that an autologous donation (when the stem cells for the injection are donated by the patient) is not necessarily safe for injection into the patient. At every step of the procedure, there is a risk for introducing infection, and cells from one part of the body may not be received well in another area.

Successful, approved stem cell treatments are confined at this point to a few procedures involving bone, skin, and eye remediation with implanted tissues. Experimental stem cell treatments that have not been through clinical trials are currently being sold to animal owners even though the treatments have insufficient evidence to support their use. It must be emphasized that sales have outpaced the science in stem cell therapy.

TONGUE-PULSE DIAGNOSIS

While standard medical procedure involves assessing the rate, regularity, and strength of an animal's pulse, alternative therapists have extended the assessment for both the pulse and the tongue, to the point that the two assessments are often paired in discussion and hyphenated when written.

Pulse diagnosis is also addressed on its own in ayurvedic assessment, where it is known as *nadi-parikha*, also transliterated as *nadi-pariksha*. Practitioners relate that they must attain an enlightened state, then use three fingers for the three Vedas while checking the pulse in order to assess physical and mental illness or imbalances.

Many acupuncturists are taught to diagnose a patient by carefully examining the tongue before giving treatment. This assessment is particularly emphasized among TCVM practitioners who are also taught pulse diagnosis, and combining these two assessments is their tongue-pulse diagnosis.

In some pulse diagnoses, the pulse is interpreted as the *vascular autonomic signal* (VAS). Some practitioners claim to be able to detect nutritional deficiencies by feeling the tonal response of the pulse, while others report they can feel the body's response to a remedy through the pulse, or VAS. Others determine what remedy to give an animal by holding a possible remedy in one hand while they check the animal's pulse with the other hand, expecting a pulse change to indicate whether or not they are holding the correct remedy.

TRADITIONAL CHINESE VETERINARY MEDICINE

Considered by many to be a whole medical system, TCVM's five main branches of study and practice are acupuncture, herbalism, nutrition therapy, qigong (or t'ai chi), and tui na. The five elements in TCVM are earth, fire, metal, water, and wood. See the earlier special review on *Acupuncture* for more information, and note the warning on TCVM in the *Supplementation* section.

TRANSCUTANEOUS ELECTRICAL NEUROMUSCULAR STIMULATION (TENS)

Also known as *Transcranial Electrical Neuro-Stimulators* (they are used on peoples' heads in migraine treatment), TENS units impart shocks through electrodes placed on the skin or through a probe. While not generally painful, the small electrical shocks can be disquieting to animals. One conventional use for the units is atrophy, where muscles waste from disuse, or paralysis, such as equine sweeney and stroke patients, especially with geriatric patients. Alternative practitioners most commonly advocate TENS for pain management.

Manufacturers of TENS units warn that the devices are not effective on pain of central origin. TENS units are never to be used on the eye, transcerebrally, or on patients with cardiac problems.

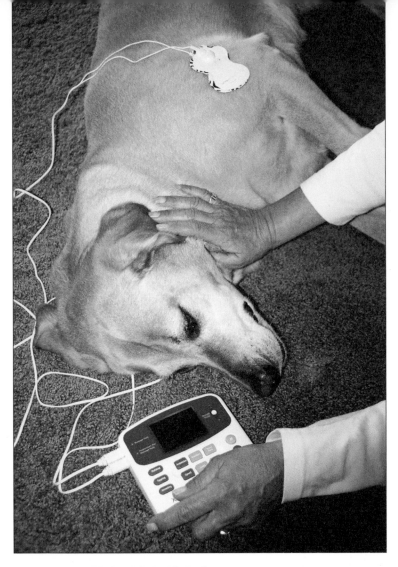

ABOVE: Will the TENS unit help this dog?

Neuromuscular electrical stimulators (NMES) are another form of the device, providing electrical stimulation of the nerves, muscles, and other tissues via the skin.

ULTRASONOGRAPHY

Ultrasound technology is an accepted diagnostic tool in mainstream medicine that has been extended to alternative uses. Also called *sonography*, an ultrasound machine transmits waves of ultra-high frequency sound into the body and records an image as the sound bounces back. Gel aids in letting the transducer glide across the animal's fur, although clipping the coat may still be necessary. Ultrasound can create a warming sensation, thus is thought to be therapeutic in that regard and often used on inflamed areas.

In 2002, the American Institute of Ultrasound in Medicine reviewed a small sample of human patients with back problems and issued an official statement the there was insufficient evidence to indicate the efficacy of ultrasonography as a treatment. The Institute's current statement, while taking no position for or against therapeutic ultrasound, warns that practitioners should be fully trained on the equipment because tissues can be damaged with ultrasound devices.

Extracorporeal shock wave therapy (ESWT) is the use of a type of ultrasound to send shock waves into the patient's body, with the hope of promoting healing in the treated area. Numerous ESWT studies have been conducted on humans and animals with results in both directions, as well as findings of damage after ESWT to tendons and ligaments. As with all treatments, be aware of factors that influence our perception of results, and know that many practitioners operate machines even though they have insufficient training.

PART 3

THE ALTERNATIVE THERAPISTS

Chiropractors, Homeopaths, Naturopaths, Holistic Vets, and More

THE DOZENS AND dozens of alternative treatments reviewed in the preceding section all have certain indications and contraindications, with varying levels of expertise behind them. But who provides these complementary and alternative treatments to the consumer's animal?

While all licensed veterinarians are medical doctors, other therapists use the title of *doctor* but are not actually medical doctors trained at an accredited medical university. These include doctors of naturopathy, doctors of homeopathy, and doctors of chiropractic. However, many veterinarians, who are schooled as conventional medical doctors, also train as naturopaths, homeopaths, and chiropractors. Some veterinarians promote their practice as holistic, and others do not. Some specialists have extensive training, and others have shockingly little. After all, anyone can purchase alternative devices, supplements, and certificates, then offer services as a practitioner. There is only one way to know what a doctor or other practitioner's individual training is: Ask.

The many hagiographic works describing founders of chiropractic, homeopathy, naturopathy, osteopathy, and other alternative medicine systems often fail to critically examine the practice. Thus, consumers can be misled by material that strictly promotes a system, and it can be difficult to get hard questions answered.

Some consumers may feel reluctant to ask practitioners about their training and experience because it can feel awkward, it seems rather forward, or they do not wish to appear distrustful. However, you, the smart consumer, are asking because you care about your animal and because you can do something with what you learn about the practitioner's education. You can make an informed choice. Do you want the practitioner to be thoroughly grounded in modern medicine? Then get a veterinarian. Do you want a vet who practices holistically? You must ask about that veterinarian's practice and ask what holistic treatment means to that vet. Do you care if your prospective practitioner has a strong medical background in addition to specific training in a type of massage? Do you even know what you want?

Just as the alternative treatments fall into certain broad categories (touch, supplementation, mystical, or other), so do the practitioners. All practitioners either do or do not define themselves as a chiropractor, homeopath, naturopath, or veterinarian. For practitioners who do not claim any of the four preceding titles, they can be considered specialists in the treatment or treatments they offer.

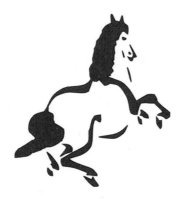

What Is a Chiropractor?

AN ANIMAL CHIROPRACTOR practices chiropractic care on animals, although the practitioner may or may not also be a veterinarian and may or may not be a chiropractor who was specially trained to work on animal patients. So what is chiropractic, and where does it come from?

Daniel David Palmer, born 1845 in Canada, self-studied medical tracts as he furthered his interest in healing. He examined the practice of using magnets and osteopathy in patient treatment and developed the idea of chiropractic—names for the Greek root words *chiro* meaning "hand" and *praxis* meaning "doing."

Palmer's concept was that misalignments or subluxations in the spine cause most disease, and he reported he had cured a man of deafness via spinal adjustment. Palmer suggested chiropractic as a treatment for everything from insanity to almost any physical disorder. As he expanded his concept, he invoked religious overtones and continued to champion the theory that the vast majority of diseases were caused by spinal misalignments. He was later convicted of practicing medicine without a license, and served a short time in jail. Palmer founded the first school for chiropractic, in Iowa.

Clearly, chiropractic originated as a school of medical thought at a time when modern medicine was still in a fledgling state and homeopathy and naturopathy were gaining ground.

It is important to recognize the difference between classical chiropractic's definition of subluxation as a misalignment causing so much disease, and the more common medical community's simpler, restricted definition: an incomplete or partial dislocation. In the conventional medical sense, a subluxation is usually acute and painful, essentially rendering the subluxated joint nearly unusable. However, chiropractors see subluxated joints as often barely out of position and still usable, with clients often unaware of the problem.

Modern chiropractors believe that bones require specific alignments for optimal function of the body and term slight changes in alignment *subluxations*, which they assert affect not only local muscles and joints but the entire nervous system as well as virtually every organ and gland of the body. Some practitioners believe that these subluxations cause or affect a broad range of diseases and disorders and consider chiropractic a whole medical system, not just a touch therapy. In addition to musculoskeletal issues such as lameness, stiffness, and poor mobility, these chiropractors may recommend chiropractic for conditions as diverse as chronic health problems, incontinence, behavioral or geriatric problems, and even seizures.

In response to legitimate criticism from science-based medicine, many modern chiropractors have modified chiropractic's dubious original foundation and recommend chiropractic treatment for musculoskeletal problems, but not for unrelated mental and physical ailments. Their treatment generally consists of manual and device-assisted manipulation of joints, most commonly the spine.

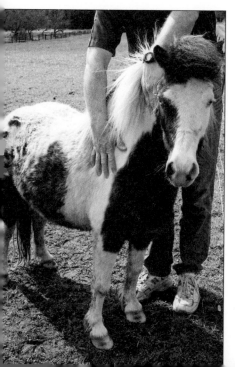

By the 1950s, animal chiropractic gained a following in the United Kingdom with John McTimoney, who adopted original chiropractic technique. In 1972, he established a chiropractic college now known as the McTimoney College of Chiropractic (formerly the Oxfordshire School of Chiropractic). The Oxford College of

LEFT: **Chiropractic has both a dubious past and a modern following, but many manual therapies are well-received by animals.**

· · 143 · ·

Equine Physical Therapy (formerly the Oxford College of Chiropractic or the Witney School of Chiropractic), teaching the McTimoney-Corley method of practice on animals, is the only other U.K. school teaching animal chiropractic.

In the late 1980s, an animal chiropractic school opened in the United States. The prestigious American Veterinary Medical Association recognized potential benefits in veterinary chiropractic in the 1990s.

Still, many veterinarians have a contentious relationship with the animal chiropractic field. Their added difficulty comes when they accuse chiropractors of practicing veterinary medicine without proper licensing or training. These vets also note that if chiropractic were in fact veterinary medicine, then chiropractic would be commonly taught in veterinary colleges.

In North America today, the American Veterinary Chiropractic Association is the largest organization accrediting animal chiropractic education and certifying animal chiropractors. For veterinarians or human chiropractors, about 150 hours' study and practicum is required to call oneself a Doctor of Chiropractic for animals. Many states and provinces have seen battles between veterinarians and chiropractors, with accusations back and forth about protecting consumers and protecting personal economic interests.

Like chiropractic for humans, animal chiropractic is not generally intended to serve as primary care but as an adjunct to conventional veterinary care. In the U.K., chiropractors cannot work without referral from a veterinarian. In Australia, only veterinarians and established chiropractors are eligible for advanced animal chiropractic training. While the United States now has several schools, and an accrediting body (the American Veterinary Chiropractic Association), chiropractic is still not generally considered the primary care system for animals but a complementary one in circumstances (such as athletic injuries or accident victims) that may especially benefit from manipulation therapy.

Animal chiropractic treatment is done via controlled manual thrusts which are intended to adjust subluxations in the vertebrae or other joints. More recently, instruments have been developed to administer these adjusting thrusts. These instruments are becoming increasingly common among practitioners. Mallets, cane ends, activators, percussors, and accelerometers are now used to make thrusts in an effort to manipulate the joint, especially on equine patients whose physical size can lead practitioners to want a mechanical advantage.

There remains considerable variation among modern animal chiropractors as to whether chiropractic is effective only for musculoskeletal problems or if chiropractic can aid behavioral problems and more. Some internationally recognized animal chiropractors disseminate scientifically inaccurate information, for example claiming all organs are innervated through the spine. Some equine chiropractors claim to treat the metabolic problem of azoturia (also called rhabdomyolosis or tying-up syndrome) with chiropractic.

While some of chiropractic's history remains an embarrassment to modern chiropractors, it may be that competent chiropractors can provide worthwhile physical therapy for some animals' musculoskeletal problems.

Although animal chiropractic treatment might be a beneficial physical therapy for some physical problems, it is not without risks, especially among senior animals or animals with degenerative bone problems.

Before seeing an animal for the first time, a chiropractor should ask the human client for a detailed history of the presenting problem. During the physical examination, chiropractors should evaluate an animal's neurological presentation—for example stiffness, weakness, or asymmetry—and pay particular attention to an animal's stance and gait. Remember that animal chiropractors are not necessarily also trained as conventional veterinarians. Chiropractors do not prescribe medicines or perform surgery.

It is important to recognize the distinction between a veterinarian who is also trained in chiropractic and someone who advertises veterinary chiropractic. The latter could refer to an animal chiropractor who is not a veterinarian, but using the term *veterinary* to indicate a practice directed at animal patients.

Chiropractic is not to be administered by untrained personnel. Manipulating an animal's spine is not without inherent risks and should never be done experimentally by people curious to try the practice on their own or other peoples' animals. The danger of injury when manipulating the spine, especially in older animals, is real. Some deaths have been attributed to chiropractic treatment, although these events are rare.

Some chiropractors are actually naturopaths, that is, they recommend and perform treatment along the same lines as would a naturopath. This can be skirting licensing requirements, unintentionally or otherwise. While laws restricting the practice of veterinary medicine to veterinarians are in place in Canada, the United States, the United Kingdom, and Australia, there is little to prevent any hobbyist from declaring himself a spinal or joint manipulator like a chiropractor and claiming to adjust animals. Competent practitioners should not hesitate to identify their training and experience when asked. Selection of a reputable animal care practitioner falls to the consumer.

Chiropractic: Adjusting Perceptions

The equine chiropractor stood on an overturned bucket at the dressage horse's hocks and pressed her hands down his spine. After a period of assessment, she began to work on him, using her fingertips and the heels of her hands to try to adjust his spine. She noted that other equine chiropractors use mallets or activators, but she is hands-on.

Next she brought out tuning forks, rang them, and applied them to places she said were acupuncture points, in order to help the horse (the primary complaint was being off in his back and poor at picking up his canter leads) heal himself. Although she wanted to see the horse for a full series of chiropractic appointments, she encouraged the owner to acquire tuning forks and continue the tuning fork follow-up.

Just any tuning fork? Applied at any point?

Well, any would work, but a fork tuned to hit middle C would work best. "It's the earth frequency," she said.

She told the owner to, "in between chiropractic appointments, apply the tuning forks along the horse's spine and at the points of his hips."

The owner thought the horse was not improved after one or two sessions and in fact seemed worse after the adjustments.

A top equestrian vet interviewed for this project became quickly exasperated when we discussed chiropractic, especially on an animal as large and powerful as a horse.

"Come on. People really think they're adjusting a horse's spine?"

I spoke to another veterinarian who came slowly to embracing chiropractic. He uses manual adjustment on many stiff horses but says it is really the horse that does the adjusting.

"They are too big and strong for us to manipulate. What happens is, I hold them in a position of flexion or extension, and as I release the hold, they put themselves into place."

He works on everything from rodeo horses to endurance athletes, jumpers to pleasure horses.

I asked if he subscribed to the foundations of chiropractic. Does he see it as a whole medical system, with the belief that minor subluxations of the spine are responsible for all medical problems?

The answer was an unequivocal no from the good doctor. He relies on the scientific medicine he learned in veterinary school. While he does share the perception that adjustments can be beneficial to certain animals, he would not recommend chiropractic for every animal.

He views chiropractic as bodywork or a manual therapy: a manipulation technique meant to encourage strained soft tissues—muscles, fascia, tendons, and ligaments—to return to their rightful position and heal.

Manual therapies, especially chiropractic, certainly have a tremendous following in both the alternative and mainstream schools of thought on rehabilitating injured animals. But assessing real improvement still requires judicious critical thinking. One chiropractor worked on a horse at a large barn when the owner was not present, but was pleased to hear the owner's report that the horse rode much better the next day. Then the practitioner realized the groom had presented her with the wrong horse. The horse reported to have ridden so much better after chiropractic had actually received no treatment at all.

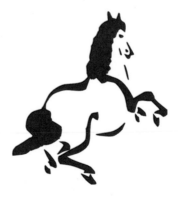

What Is a Homeopath?

A VETERINARY HOMEOPATH is a practitioner who practices homeopathy on animals, although the practitioner may or may not also be a qualified veterinarian. So what is homeopathy, and where does it come from?

Christian Friedrich Samuel Hahnemann, born 1755 in Germany, was a medical doctor and translator who developed the concept of homeopathy—named for the Greek root words *homo* meaning "same" and *pathos* meaning "disease"—as a unique approach to medicine. Medicine in his time was indeed an often barbaric proposition with an unimpressive record of success due to poor hygiene and the lack of understanding about physiology and pathology.

Materia Medica is an old Latin term for the body of knowledge about medical material or medical treatments. (A first-century Greek text also bore the title *Materia Medica*, as had numerous others.) While translating William Cullen's *Materia Medica* into German, Hahnemann noticed the text indicated cinchona bark was used to treat malaria fever, and he reportedly ingested some of the bark and felt he developed malarial symptoms within a few weeks.

Cinchona, a tree or shrub with about twenty-five varieties, is found throughout South America and had long been used as a folk medicine. Quinine kills the mosquito-borne parasite that causes malaria, and the quinine alkaloid occurs naturally in many plants, including cinchonas. However, Hahnemann concluded that cinchona gave him malarial symptoms and then concluded that a substance that causes symptoms in a healthy person would cure the same symptom in an unhealthy person.

Curing through similars was a concept pursued by ancient Greeks as well. It contrasted strongly with the idea of curing through anti-dotes, substances that fought a problem. The term *allopathy—allo* meaning "other"—now sometimes used as a pejorative reference for mainstream medicine, originally sprung up as a homeopathic term for what was then modern medicine.

LAWS OF HOMEOPATHY

Hahnemann coined the term *similia similibus curantur*, also known as letting *like cure like*, or the *law of similars*. He carried on his hypothesis with the notion that a substance becomes more powerful the more the dose is diluted (law of infinitesimalism) and developed a system of shaking and diluting substances in alcohol, water, or both (law of potentization), then tested his concoctions. Because he believed substances that caused a particular symptom in a healthy person would cure a sick person with the same symptoms, he tested substances on himself and others, detailing how people felt when administered the substance (law of proving).

SUCCUSSION

Hahnemann crafted homeopathic remedies with vigorous succussion (shaking) between dilutions and worked hard to determine exactly how long a mixture should be succussed and then left to stand between dilutions. He particularly promoted succussing by striking the vial of solution against a leather-bound book.

DILUTION

Creating the common 30c homeopathic remedy of arnica, for example, consists of crushing the arnica flowers, leaves, stems, and roots and soaking the plant parts in a mixture of 90 percent alcohol and 10 percent water. After this base has been shaken and allowed to steep, it is strained into a dark bottle, creating a tincture. One drop of this tincture is combined with ninety-nine drops of alcohol or water and shaken—this is its first dilution. Next, one drop of that diluted solution is again combined with ninety-nine drops of alcohol (or water). Repeating the 1:99 dilution—one drop of the last dilution to 99 more drops of water or alcohol—a total of thirty times yields the homeopathic dilution noted as 30c, which is perhaps the most common dilution sold.

The remedies are usually created in their commercial form by placing a few drops of the last dilution in a jar of lactose pills. While it may seem a concern that not all of those sugar pills definitely receive some of the final dilution solution, the final solution actually does not have any of the original herbal remedy anyway.

A 200c solution, considered by homeopaths to be stronger than 30c even though the 200c remedies are put through two hundred repetitions of the 1:99 dilution cycle, may be restricted to professional homeopathic use and is not readily available.

There are also x dilutions, in which one drop of the original tea is mixed with nine drops of diluting water or alcohol, then one drop of that resulting solution is mixed with nine drops of dilutant (it is now a 2x strength solution). A 12x remedy has gone through twelve repetitions of the 1:9 dilution cycle.

Contemporary homeopathic remedies are commonly sold in health food stores and recommended by homeopaths, naturopaths, and numerous holistic veterinarians. The remedies are manufactured with original plant, animal, and mineral parts.

In her August 16, 2003, open letter to peers regarding the Vaccine-Serum-Toxin Act of 1913 in relation to homeopathy, veterinarian Gloria Dodd notes that she uses 30c homeopathic nosodes, which have none of the original physical substance, but are instead just "pure energy" (http://www.cavm.net/Files/Dodd.htm).

Indeed Avogadro's number (6.02x10 to the twenty-third power)—the numerical constant estimated by Johann Josef Loschmidt to count the particles in a

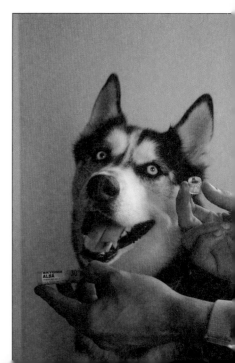

RIGHT: **It is important to understand the dilution of homeopathic remedies.**

· · 151 · ·

substance—indicates that at homeopathic dilutions (beyond the 12c dilution), none of the original substance remains in the final product.

The U.K. Parliament published a report on the evidence for homeopathy in 2010, which concluded that the British National Health Service should not fund homeopathy.

ADDITIONAL WORK

In the 1830s, Hahnemann produced his own materia medica, calling it the *Materia Medica Pura* and listing all substances that had met his provings. One modern version of the text is called the *Homeopathic Pharmacopoeia of the United States*. Hahnemann's *Organon der rationellen Heilkunde* (translated to *Organon of the Healing Art*) is still the classic homeopathic text. In the book, pages are devoted to listing symptoms that may be cured. Some of these symptoms, such as falling asleep while reading, are not applicable to veterinary applications, but many can transfer to animals (such as trembling near females, or yawning and stretching). He later noticed some of his patients did not remain cured of symptoms after his treatment and developed the theory that three different miasms—psora, syphilis and gonorrhea—caused all disease.

VETERINARY HOMEOPATHY

Baron Clemens Maria Franz von Bönninghausen, a contemporary of Hahnemann's, wrote extensively on homeopathy and is often credited as being the first to extend homeopathy to animal care. Veterinary homeopathy is practiced in various forms throughout much of the world today, with associations in the U.K., the United States, Australia, and beyond.

As noted, in the early 1900s, rapid advances in modern medicine turned many scientists and consumers away from fields such as chiropractic, naturopathy, and homeopathy; however homeopathy received some legal sanctioning initiated by U.S. Senator Royal Samuel Copeland.

Copeland, a homeopathic physician, was instrumental in the passage of the 1938 Food, Drug, and Cosmetic Act, which, among many other things, recognized the profession of homeopathy. While the profession is recognized, the remedies do not have to demonstrate effectiveness to the Food and Drug Administration in the way that is required of conventional drugs.

Modern homeopaths who understand the calculation of molecular presence with Avogadro's number (thus recognizing that none of the original substance remains after so much dilution) still claim homeopathy works and theorize the following reasons for why it works: the memory of the original substance remains to impart treatment; an electromagnetic state is achieved in the creation of the remedy and magnetite in animal's brains is sensitive to the remedy; water used in the mixture has stored energy that heals; or, cure is explained by chaos theory, because small changes can have enormous results. Modern critics of homeopathy attribute any improvement to the placebo response.

Modern veterinary homeopaths see three response possibilities for any type of treatment: palliation, suppression, or cure, with cure, not alleviation of symptoms, being the goal of the homeopathic system of treatment.

Although they are generally quite safe to use—being essentially inert—because homeopathic remedies sold in the form of little milk-sugar pellets without any original botanical substance, they should not be given to animals with lactose intolerance. Practitioners warn that the pills should not be touched by the person administering them and generally should not be combined with other remedies.

Remember the distinction between veterinarians who practice homeopathy and a homeopath who practices on animals, that is, not all homeopaths who practice on animals are also qualified veterinarians. Advocates for homeopathic treatment for animals have asserted that when the treated animal's symptoms appear to be getting worse, it does not mean that the animal really is getting worse.

The Academy of Veterinary Homeopathy has a referral list and provides suggestions on what to ask a homeopathic veterinarian to decide if the vet is practicing classical homeopathy and admonishes that more than one therapy should not be given to an animal at a time, as acupuncture, chiropractic, or even an allopathic ear ointment, for example, interferes with an animal's response to the homeopathic treatment.

The American Holistic Veterinary Medical Association also lists practitioners who use homeopathy and has this to say about the treatments: "Homeopathic remedies contain vibrational energy essences that match the patterns present in the diseased state within the ailing patient."

Modern homeopaths who treat animals may employ a host of alternative diagnostic treatments covered in this book, from radionics to electrodermal testing, but homeopathic remedies and their hallmark ultra-dilutions remain the cornerstone of homeopathy.

Legal regulation and recognition of homeopaths who are not veterinarians varies from region to region. Selection of a reputable animal care practitioner falls to the consumer.

Pain in the Gut: Homeopathic Ulcer Treatment

Ulcers in horses seem to be on the rise. A generation ago, horse owners heard little about ulcers. Now, glossy general magazines for the horsey set frequently include advertisements for treatment of equine gastric ulcer syndrome (EGUS). Ulcer prevention plans receive regular coverage in those magazines' articles.

Ulcers are definitively diagnosed via endoscopy, an expensive procedure. The average veterinarian does not possess an endoscope (an instrument that is passed through a horse's mouth and esophagus into his stomach to allow the administrator to view the stomach lining on a monitor). Not equipped to perform definitive diagnosis, vets commonly diagnose ulcers as a best guess, after a careful examination that includes observation, asking about behavioral symptoms, and eliciting a complete history from the owner or rider.

Veterinarians often treat suspected ulcers empirically, that is, they prescribe a drug used to treat ulcers, such as cimetidine or ranitidine hydrochloride, and if the horse seems to improve, then the improvement is taken as confirmation that the horse has, or had, an ulcer. Horse off their feed or showing behavioral signs of irritation often become better eaters or more manageable after ulcer drug treatment, which of course does not mean that the improvement is due to the treatment—an animal may have improved in its cooperation with training, or there could be another factor in improved appetite or manageability.

Another modern ulcer treatment for horses is administered daily for a month, at a cost of about forty dollars a day. This expense makes the empirical treatment with ranitidine attractive to many vet and clients.

Some vets are now using an alternative treatment, something faster and cheaper. I talked to one of these veterinarians who sees quite a few horses he believes suffer from ulcers.

"I used to put horses on ranitidine for ten days or two weeks and see if their appetite came back, if they were less snotty, less cinchy."

Cinchy, or girthy, horses are those who act irritated, upset, or fussy when saddled, especially when the cinch or girth is tightened.

This vet now uses a homeopathic ulcer treatment and advises he's seen horses turn around in just three days. It's hard to argue with results.

"What's in it?"

"Aloe," he told me. "And some herbs."

"And it's actually at homeopathic dilution?" (See *What Is a Homeopath?* for detail on the extreme dilution of homeopathic remedies.)

He hesitated. "I don't know. I get it from this other veterinarian. He mixes it up himself." But he advised that he not only treats ulcers with this homeopathic preparation, he prevents them.

What Is a Naturopath?

A NATUROPATH IS a practitioner who practices naturopathy, a system of treatment that champions the body's natural healing abilities, and eschews drugs and surgical intervention. The term *naturopathy* is taken from Greek and Latin roots that mean, in combination, "natural disease." While misnamed, the founding tenets of naturopathy are reflected in the concept of emphasizing nature and the body's natural healing mechanisms.

Although naturopathy was practiced by others, German immigrant Benedict Lust established it in the United States by the 1800s. In Europe, Lust had been a patient and then a student of Father Sebastian Kneipp, who promoted cure via nature: a belief that healthy food, sunshine, and exercise—with hydrotherapy as a treatment—were the way to healing.

By the early 1900s, numerous schools of naturopathic medicine opened in Canada and the United States. Rapid advances in modern medicine negatively impacted the naturopathy movement. Today,

BELOW: Rehabilitation through physical exercise such as swimming is widely accepted, while a belief in naturopathic healing due to immersion's curative power is not.

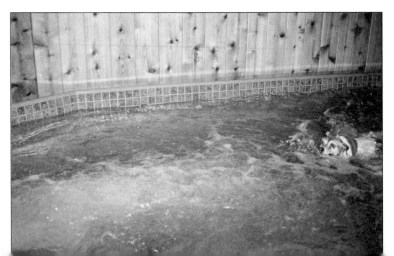

there are a number of naturopathic colleges in the United States (examples are: Southwest College of Naturopathic Medicine and Health Sciences in Tempe, Arizona; Bastyr University in Kenmore, Washington; National College of Natural Medicine in Portland, Oregon; University of Bridgeport College of Naturopathic Medicine in Bridgeport, Connecticut, and the National University of Health Sciences in Lombard, Illinois) and in Canada (Canadian College of Naturopathic Medicine in North York, Ontario), but none of these specifically teach animal naturopathy.

There is much to be said for turning to healthy living as a path to health. Veterinarians (and medical doctors for humans) see countless patients for a variety of lifestyle illnesses as well as other problems exacerbated by unhealthy living choices. These patients would be greatly helped if their owners fed them, engaged them, and exercised them more wisely. An overweight dog suffering from joint problems would simply be a happier animal at a healthy weight, and an owner who turns to conventional veterinarians or alternative practitioners without addressing the obvious weight problem is being unrealistic.

It must also be noted that acknowledging the body's innate ability to cure itself is something conventional medicine certainly recognizes. Veterinarians do not think that they cure a laceration, but they understand that the body regenerates. Thus, naturopathy's unique feature is not really the recognition of the body's ability to heal but rather the philosophical rejection of surgery and advanced pharmaceutical intervention.

Veterinary naturopathy is practiced today by veterinarians who have pursued the subject, by naturopaths who have pursued the study and treatment of animal patients, and even by practitioners who have not studied a formal curriculum of naturopathy or veterinary medicine.

Foundations of classical naturopathy include herbology, nutrition therapy, cold and hot hydrotherapy, and exposure to fresh air and sunlight. It is a school of care that shuns synthetic drugs. The healing power of nature—known in Latin as *vis medicatrix naturae*—remains the founding principle of naturopathy, for animals or otherwise.

NATUROPATHY AND DRUGS

In noting that naturopathy avoids drug treatment, we struggle again to correctly define terms. Many naturopaths employ homeopathic remedies. While many practitioners consider these remedies to be drugs, they find them acceptable to administer and recommend, but naturopaths are unlikely to support conventional modern pharmaceutical therapy.

VETERINARY NATUROPATHY METHODS

Patient assessment, diagnosis, and treatment from naturopaths is as varied as the practitioners. Modern naturopaths for animals may attempt to assess and diagnose patients through kinesiology, iridology, electrodermal testing, radionics, reflexology, or by other means.

Treatment may be through classical fasting, soaking, and exercise, or may also venture into homeopathy and other alternative therapies such as detoxification cleanses.

Always, veterinary naturopathy emphasizes client education to establish healthy living conditions for the animal. Prevention of illness is key.

Some principles of naturopathy are not unique when compared to other medical systems, but they are good ideas: The doctor is a teacher, the doctor should do no harm to the patient, healthy living prevents many medical complaints, the whole patient should be treated, and the real cause of the disease should be identified then treated, rather than merely treating symptoms.

The American Veterinary Naturopathic Association advises the naturopathic approach is less costly than conventional care.

Remember that naturopaths who treat animals may be veterinarians with an interest in naturopathy, may be naturopaths with an interest in animals, or may not be qualified at all. Selection of a reputable animal care practitioner falls to the consumer.

What Is a Holistic Veterinarian?

A HOLISTIC VETERINARIAN is a veterinarian who treats the animal from a holistic approach, that is, considering the whole body and causative factors in the presenting condition—such as diet, exercise, and living situation—to include the animal's mental health.

Note that being a holistic veterinarian does not inherently mean that the veterinarian subscribes to any alternative treatments. Strictly speaking, with the exception of veterinarians who become specialists in a narrow field, all practicing veterinarians were taught to be and should be, holistic in their approach. It is a foundation of good general health care that diet, exercise, and lifestyle are considered. Indeed any conventional veterinarian might understandably bristle at the comment that their training "looks at the most specific, minute part of an individual, and loses sight of the individual as a whole" (Schwartz, page vi).

It would be far more difficult to find a veterinarian who actually claims not to treat animals holistically than it is to find vets who advertise their practice as giving holistic care. The reality is that the term *holistic* has become another buzzword, with an unspoken understanding that many veterinarians who label themselves holistic vets are veterinarians who integrate alternative diagnostics and/or treatments into their services, and perhaps only practice alternative medicine, having abandoned their original science-based medical training.

While there are organizations for holistic veterinarians and other holistic animal care groups, there is no simple determinant or certifying organization that deems one veterinarian a holistic vet as compared to a traditional, mainstream, or conventional veterinarian.

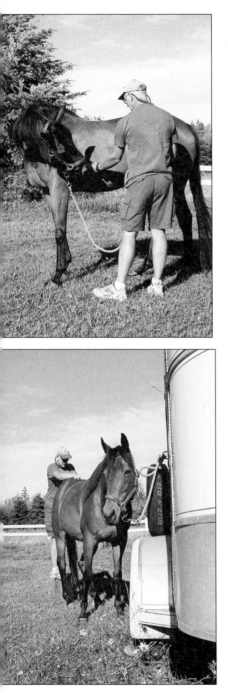

LEFT: **Holistic care is considered by all good veterinarians. This spinal exam includes checking for flexion . . .**

This understood, what do good holistic veterinarians do? They examine everything about the animal. Starting with the animal's diet, for example, they teach their clients to compare premium foods with warehouse store brands. (Learning to understand product labels is a must for conscientious owners.) Holistic vets consider the whole animal and the animal's whole situation. And they may well be more likely to embrace some alternative methods than veterinarians who do not specifically promote their practice as holistic.

It is certainly true that many conventional veterinarians eschew all or a great deal of alternative medicine, so clients who want to consider alternatives often turn to veterinarians who advertise having a holistic practice.

The American Holistic Veterinary Medical Association notes the following holistic modalities: acupuncture, behavior modification, chiropractic, herbal medicine, homeopathy, mega nutrients and augmentation therapy, nutritional therapy, traditional Chinese veterinary medicine, and other modalities of diagnosis and therapy.

LEFT: **. . . as well as symmetry.**

What are these *other modalities*? Their referral list notes—in addition to conventional medicine—the following specialties:

Primary AHVMA Specialties
Acupuncture
Aromatherapy
Chiropractic
Flower Essences
Herbal Medicine
Homeopathy
Low-Level Laser Therapy
Mega-Nutrient Therapy
Nutritional Therapy
Osteopathy
Rehabilitation and Sports Medicine
Stem Cell Therapy

It must be emphasized that being a solid holistic veterinarian does not mean that the vet must embrace any of these treatments. A holistic approach demands the vet consider the animal's physical and mental living situation, its diet and exercise, all of its symptoms and complaints, its genetics and potential, as well as its handler's skills when evaluating the animal and its presenting condition.

Having a holistic outlook does not necessarily demand the veterinarian believe in any mystical practices, employ unproven treatment methods, or engage every new fad or revived bit of classical folk medicine. A holistic approach to a sore-backed horse (or even many lameness issues and other strains), for example, includes examining the horse's tack and work. Certainly not every veterinarian who practices holistically is a member of the AHVMA or a similar organization in another country.

VACCINATION

Some holistic veterinarians have a very different approach to vaccination than conventional vets. However, using nosodes and titer tests in place of modern vaccination simply will not afford animals the same level of protection against communicable diseases. Still, anti-vaccination groups make a fair point when they decry overvaccination. Any vaccination an animal receives should be because the animal is at a reasonable risk of exposure, not because the veterinarian wished to see the animal for an annual examination as is infamously noted in a major veterinary text.

Again, finding a veterinarian claiming to be holistic isn't particularly difficult, but finding one who claims *not* to be holistic would be a challenge. Veterinarians are trained to consider causative factors when making a patient assessment. Other than specialists, who may restrict their practice to one aspect of care—for instance a veterinary surgeon specializing in orthopedics, who may specialize further still in one area, such as knees, for example—all veterinarians are trained to consider a patient holistically rather than merely examining one presenting symptom, such as a skin condition.

Some do a better job than others at this holistic approach. Assessing what a particular veterinarian believes and offers is the client's job. Selection of a reputable animal care practitioner falls to the consumer.

Holistic Health: Da

This great-grandson of a Preakness winner was adopted at age twelve to his final home. Although his stellar lineage was such that he had been nominated for the Breeders' Cup, his racing career didn't pan out. He seemed off in his back and was given away, and then leased out. Eventually he wound up two hundred pounds underweight, unhappy, and untrusting in a rescue shelter. The shelter called him Da and identified him explicitly as a light riding horse, with wobbler's syndrome.

The man who adopted the horse affectionately called him the Doo-Da.

Da had issues. He twisted his mouth and head in obvious stress behavior when separated from familiar surroundings. When mounted, he sometimes abruptly dropped one hip several inches. He was girthy and resistant to taking the bit, pinning his ears even though he was handled gently. He also exhibited stringhalt signs, sometimes suddenly snapping one hind leg to his belly and standing still, looking stressed. Stringhalt is uncommon, and bilateral stringhalt even more so, but Da was bilateral. When made to stand on the hind leg that he had been holding to his belly, he snapped his other hind leg up and held it.

One vet said the horse's knee was locking and suggested a surgical knee-release procedure. She referred the client to the best equine hospital within several hundred miles. There, the head veterinary surgeon pointed out that the knee doesn't lock in flexion. Da didn't happen to exhibit his stringhalt on the day he was examined at the elite hospital. The surgeon thought the shelter vet's diagnosis of wobbler's might have been correct, but expensive testing would be needed to confirm this. Given that the horse's job was light trail riding, there wasn't much to be done for his being occasionally off in the hind end.

Another veterinarian who advertised a holistic practice prescribed homeopathic remedies and was either unwilling or unable to explain the meaning of the letter C in the 30c dosage arnica prescription. The vet rented out a laser unit, suggested magnets and recommended chiropractic adjustments. The horse put up with acupuncture, chiropractic, and other remedies with the same long-suffering attitude he exhibited when symptomatic with his hind fetlock held up to his abdomen. There was no consistent pattern to what brought on his stringhalt.

Clearly, Da didn't enjoy chiropractic, acupuncture, magnets, or lasers. Because the horse was not a good candidate for trying additional nontraditional treatments, because there were too many unanswered critical questions, his owner canceled further alternative sessions and located a solid equine veterinarian.

This vet applauded the horse's home, light riding use, feeding program, routine care for his hooves and teeth, and schedule of preventative care, including vaccinations, worming, and examinations.

Da obviously did enjoy a good home with good pasture and a pasture mate. He became more and more manageable under consistent, gentle handling.

Over time, the horse called The Doo-Da gained weight, tone, and trust. He became a beautiful, dutiful fellow and is a happy senior enjoying trail rides, especially if they offer a good view. For years, he exhibited no stringhalt signs, and he led green horses down mountain trails and across streams. Holistic care—good nutrition, comfortable shelter, a pasture mate, essentially no negative stress, good routine health maintenance, and the nice job of light-duty trail riding—healed this horse.

It is worth noting that the vet who offered no alternative treatments nor advertised himself as a holistic veterinarian did in fact treat Da holistically. He treated the whole animal, as do all good general veterinarians.

Ten years later, Da again suddenly had bilateral stringhalt. Out came his general veterinarian who found and relieved a small toe abscess. The vet predicted the stringhalt would resolve spontaneously, and it was indeed gone by that afternoon.

Who Are the Specialists?

AN ASTOUNDING NUMBER of practitioners offering alternative treatments for animals are not veterinarians, nor are they chiropractors, homeopaths, or naturopaths. They are massage therapists and consultants and other private practitioners who specialize in one or numerous alternative treatments.

The alphabet soup after practitioners' names can be confusing or impressive. By convention, some abbreviations for degrees or certifications are listed in various orders, sometimes with and sometimes without periods after the letter, although there is generally no formal standard for how degrees, diplomas, and course completions are

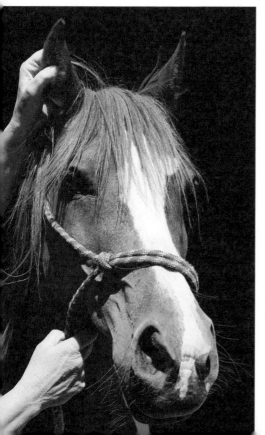

LEFT: Independent practitioners offer everything from auriculotherapy to zone therapy.

denoted. Consider this partial list of abbreviations indicating specialized training or services offered by a practitioner:

AT	aromatherapist
CA	certified aromatherapist
CAC	certified animal chiropractor
CAT	certified aquatic therapist
CBW	canine body worker
CEMT	certified equine massage therapist
CHT	certified hyperbaric technologist
CVCP	certified veterinary chiropractor
CVH	certified veterinary herbalist
CVHE	certified veterinary herbalist educator
DC	doctor of chiropractic
Dipl. ACVH	diplomate in American College of Veterinary Herbalists
DH	doctor of homeopathy
DHM	doctor of homeopathic medicine
DN	doctor of naturopathy
DVetHom	diploma in veterinary homeopathy
DVM	doctor of veterinary medicine
EBW	equine body worker
EMT	equine massage therapist
L.Ac.	licensed acupuncturist
LAMP	large animal massage practitioner
LMP	licensed massage practitioner
MEBW	master equine body worker
MT	massage therapist
MTC	manual therapist certified
ND	naturopathic doctor
PT	physical therapist
RM	reiki master
SAMP	small animal massage practitioner
WC	wellness consultant

As has been demonstrated in the review of alternative treatments, the therapies in which these practitioners specialize also offer an array of abbreviations. It is important to determine whether an alternative practitioner has direct training and experience with animals. Not everybody realizes that a dog's hock is roughly equivalent to a person's heel. Not all knowledge and treatments transfer well between the species.

CERTIFICATION

In researching alternative therapeutic modalities and the quality of evidence and education behind them, the author encountered both a correspondence course in equine aromatherapy expected to take six months to a year for completion and special canine or equine massage courses—conducted mostly online—that suggested one could start a business as a practitioner after a five-day course. A startling number of entrepreneurs certify others in their personal brand of alternative treatment. Many courses finish with the granting of a *certificate of completion*, allowing graduated students to honestly advertise themselves as certified at the treatment.

A specialist promoting an education as a certified acupuncturist, myotherapist, herbalist, communicator, or any other specialty has not really given the consumer much information. In order to evaluate the services offered by any practitioner, one must ask serious questions about the person's training, education, and practice. Some have a four-year degree; some have trained for less than a week. Certainly, to obtain a bachelor of science in equine studies with a concentration in equine therapy is to apply significant time and dedication to the pursuit of knowledge, but the consumer must ask about more than the length of the specialist's study (see the section on *How and When to Choose Alternative Treatment*).

Licensed practitioner is a phrase many alternative therapists advertise. It could merely mean that the practitioner has paid a small fee to the local government for a business license. There may be a licensing board—and several certifying or accrediting organizations—for the field in which the specialist works—but the practitioner may not have met the criteria for any of these organizations. Who certified or licensed the practitioner? After how much study? Again, ask and research what you learn.

Independent practitioner generally means that the therapist is not a doctor of veterinary medicine, or advertising qualification as a naturopath, chiropractor, or homeopath. The person is usually operating independently of a supervising medical authority or regulation. While this is not necessarily a bad thing, it should provoke more questions.

Practitioners who appear equivocal about relating their training may have a reason for their ambiguity or reluctance. Ask again. A business card and a professional-looking color brochure about a therapist's practice, endorsed by an international association of that therapy, becomes much less impressive upon scrutiny if a second look reveals the practitioner is the founder and sole member of the organization.

Many companies sell alternative therapeutic devices and goods, including publications and educational services, as well as teach clinics. A person may take a one-day clinic in using a cold laser device, tuning forks, a qigong massage machine, or a chiropractic mallet, for example, and then be given a certificate of attendance by the clinic provider. The student then might advertise certification in using the device and begin providing services.

Specialists' businesses can build out of surprisingly small startups. A tip sheet for someone wishing to commence a career from very little would suggest adapting, twisting, or combining a folk remedy with a manual therapy and perhaps a belief in a special energy system. Next, create several levels of training for new practitioners. Consider creating an international certifying organization as well.

What can specialists and other alternative practitioners really do for our good animals? There is no doubt that devoted students and therapists can amass a great deal of valuable and provocative information. There is, of course, a wide variety of alternative treatments for these specialists to engage in: touch therapies, some form of supplementation, methods that are mystical in nature, or something else entirely. Certainly, there are some skilled therapists who are not doctors but who have a track record of success at treating animals.

In the United States, laws vary tremendously from state to state as to whether an animal massage therapist, for example, may practice without direct, immediate supervision by a veterinarian. Some states allow massage freely, some have unclear laws on the subject, some restrict the practice to veterinarians, while still others allow veterinary technicians to perform animal massage. This legal spectrum may contribute to the creation of so many bodywork and touch treatments that are advertised as *different* from simple massage. If the practitioner is not claiming to be a massage therapist, then the practitioner is not subject to laws restricting massage therapy.

Clearly, there are dozens of repetitions in remedies and therapies. Separating the snake oil from the useful can be overwhelming. Practitioners are often competing for the consumers' dollars and may be turf-guarding while promoting their treatment above another. Alternatively, they may be working together, supporting others' work, with animals' best interests sincerely in mind.

Not all alternative treatments are explored in this review. (What about detoxification treatment, electuary, equine neuromuscular technique, geomancy, Hoppe method, orthopedic mobilization, polarity therapy, raindrop, TAT, and dozens of other methods, theories, and practices on the offer in the realm of alternative treatments?) New permutations of alternative treatments are constantly being defined, refined, and made up. Some specialists create new terms as a means of skirting laws meant to restrict lay practitioners. For example, if they are not legally allowed to assess a problem, they coin a virtual synonym for the problem, say X, and advise they can detect X. It is important to verify a practitioner's scope of practice. Legislation such as the Healthcare Truth and Transparency Act of 2007 has not diminished the consumer's responsibility to ask about specialists' training and abilities.

Prescription medications require a veterinarian's signature for purchase, yet non-veterinarian practitioners have begun writing "prescriptions" (recommendations) of their own for substances found in catalogs, on the Internet, in the garden, the grocery store, health food stores, and other retail outlets. This leaves real questions about the safety of these practices. If an alternative practitioner prescribes a particular physical therapy for a dog or a particular angle for a horse's hooves and the animal suffers, who is responsible?

Because you care for your animal, you are ultimately responsible. Recognize the limits and capabilities of the many specialists who provide alternative treatments. Selection of a reputable animal care practitioner falls to the consumer.

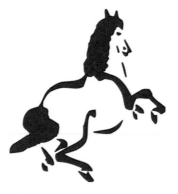

PART 4

IT'S YOUR CHOICE

How and When to Choose Alternative Treatments

FOR A HOST of reasons, people are making active, specific, and personal choices about their animals' care. While this interest can only be a good thing, the result can be less than positive when people make uninformed decisions. Alternative treatments run the large spectrum from foolish to fundamental. There are risks involved with ill-considered forays into mystical, supplemental, touch, and other therapies.

Consumers would do well to make a significant effort to learn about the available options.

The methods used for exploring alternative treatments must be sound. With inadequate investigation and casual selection from among the many options, time and money can easily be wasted. Worse, the animal may suffer needlessly. It is important to make a careful, considered investigation and, subsequently, equally thoughtful decisions about animal care.

At first blush, one consumer may want a holistic vet who does iridology. Another decides to find a homeopath or naturopath who uses comfrey. Someone else seeks a chiropractor who works classically, without a mallet. Another person thinks classical adjustments are too slow and a tool must be used. Yet another might look for a practitioner who uses all the latest trends, every new cold laser and other devices, body mapping and massage technique combined with mystical aspects. Or perhaps someone has a friend who had a good experience with acupressure and now recommends it to everyone and their good dogs.

There is no explicit rubric for making these choices, but learning all one can about the options available is an excellent start. More information is not much further away than simply formulating the questions. Before even turning to alternative care, it makes sense to be grounded in good conventional care. And the first questions to be asked should be directed to us, the consumers. How and when do we choose alternatives? Let's break the question into two parts and first examine how.

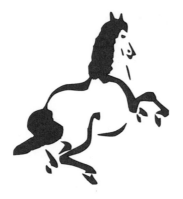

How to Choose Alternatives for Your Animal

QUESTIONS TO ASK Yourself When Considering an Alternative Treatment

Does Your Veterinarian Echo Your Views on Animal Care?

Locating a vet who shares your values in this regard only makes sense. Implicit in this advice is that people must first determine their own values. Also, it is not necessary to find someone who completely agrees with you—a professional who accommodates your views on animal care is all that is needed. After all, this keeps you from having a yes-man on your team. Flexibility is important in working with animals in any case, and medical issues tend to require adjustment in how they are approached. If you are unhappy with your vet, ask yourself why, and be sure to identify a valid explanation for your concerns.

Are You Doing All You Can for Your Animal with Respect to a Healthy Lifestyle?

Don't turn to a treatment just to make up for a failure to provide good, preventative health care. Prevention being the first line of defense, recognize the essential keys to vibrant physical health: genetics, nutrition, exercise, a good living situation. The latter especially affects an animal's mental health and includes the provision of positive stimulation while keeping negative stress at a minimum. Regarding the first factor, genetics, don't breed or be party to supporting ill-bred animals. The two remaining factors—nutrition and exercise—are also a matter of managing the animal's life with informed decisions regarding the animal's care. Providing a well-bred animal with a healthy living situation that includes good nutrition and appropriate exercise handles the bulk of preventative health care. The immune system does not function optimally when an animal is not at its healthiest.

It is important to stay current on findings. Consider animal feed and the fluctuations it has experienced. Propylene glycol and benzoates were initially permitted in commercial dog foods but are no longer allowed, as they were found to be unsafe. In 2007, large-scale pet food contamination resulted in the recall of many cat and dog foods thought to have been safe, and many pet deaths were attributed to the contamination.

Further, nutritional needs of an animal change with age and workload, and good nutrition is a matter of science, not speculation. For example, a person might intuitively think an all-meat diet is appropriate for a dog, but such a diet is actually unhealthy and incomplete. Review your feeding program with a competent veterinarian to be sure your animal is receiving proper nutrition.

Regarding parasite control, like weeds in the garden, they too are best dealt with by prevention. Let's take as an example, the family dog. Because you're paying attention to the dog's environment (physical and mental) and diet, the pooch is well placed to deal with these pests. But contact with other peoples' animals can introduce fleas, ticks, worms, and other parasites. Consider every facet of health when building your animal's good lifestyle. Remember, the best health program is based on healthy living as a preventative to disease, which must include a good diet, good exercise, and mental stimulation in a pleasant, stress-free living situation.

Why Do You Want to Try This Alternative Treatment?

It is important to identify *why* you think this treatment will do what you hope it will do. Be clear with yourself about what you hope to achieve and consciously recognize whether or not it is a reasonable goal. Think about some of the other common reasons people give when they decide to try an alternative treatment:

Why? I don't know . . .

This is not much of an answer. Force yourself to articulate your reasons, and if they aren't very solid, get better reasons. It's fine to have a valid explanation for disagreeing with your veterinarian, or to change practitioners completely, but do have good reasons.

- *Because So-and-So, an elite in the discipline in which I compete my animal, uses a Siberian ginseng and wu wei zi formula.*

Emulating the pros has its merits in many aspects of caring for or competing with animals. But don't assume anyone using a product has done the smart consumer research. Check it out yourself with a good critical review.

- *Because the winner of the championship is in a magazine advertisement with a quote about how the dog's performance was enhanced with this supplement.*

Remember, an elite competitor who is receiving sponsorship dollars to be photographed and make a promotional recommendation on an herbal combination is far from a critical appraisal of the producers' claims for their product.

- *Because the literature in and on the package says it can cure my dog's allergy. The package says this product improves the dog's vitality. The flyer claims this treatment heals the horse's wound faster.*

When the literature is stating an unproven claim as fact, it is already misleading. This is a recurring problem in promotional literature and misstated advice by practitioners promoting their treatments. Be a mindful listener and a critical reader. Recognize when opinion or belief is being stated as fact. The material must be viewed suspiciously when opinions are misrepresented. Praise from a sales representative is an unconvincing compliment. When reviewing promotional material, whether in person, on a website, or with direct literature, consider the motives of the person dispensing the advertising. And do consider it advertising, not pure, objective information.

- *Because my friend suggested it.*

Whatever sparks your interest in an alternative treatment, do the smart work of research and critical evaluation of what you learn, keeping your conventional veterinarian in the loop and evaluating the vet's input. It's fairly easy to find and read information persuasive in favor of the alternative, but it's important to see the other side. Actively seek the contrasting opinion in addition to finding recommendations on the therapy and specific therapists.

For smart consumers who have a good vet, follow a strong preventative health care program, provide their animals with a healthy lifestyle, and have elected to try alternative treatment for articulate reasons, there is first a research path to take.

Doing the Research

Use the standard research tools of referrals, organizations, libraries, electronic databases, and the Internet. The reference section of this book lists numerous primary organizations. A bounty of resources awaits the interested consumer of information.

Considerable investment has been made on alternative treatments for human patients; availing oneself of that information makes a good starting point. From the United Kingdom comes the Cochrane Collaboration (www.thecochranelibrary.com), with over ten thousand volunteers from nearly one hundred countries reviewing biomedical tests of all sorts. At worthy websites such as The Cochrane Library or sciencebasedmedicine.org, one need only click, read, and learn. The sites offer basic and advanced search functions to home in on the topic of interest.

Recognize careless literature while studying. Frequently, causation is declared or implied when it has not been actually demonstrated. For example, a statement such as "I gave him X herb formula and then his swelling/coughing/lethargy improved right away" implies that the treatment cured the animal. This is an example of a study in which there was no control, no blinding, no randomization, and a sample size of one subject! All that is really known is that the treatment was given and that the animal got better, but a definite link between the two events is not known—the animal may well have improved without whatever remedy the caregiver offered.

With a careful reading, every book, flyer, and web page offers suggestions for further research. Remember, metaphysical claims are inherently unprovable. Understand this while recognizing pseudoscience. Employ critical thinking, approaching each therapy from two routes: a willingness to believe and a healthy skepticism.

BE A CRITICAL READER

There is a great deal of conflicting advice available. One report may debunk a therapy while another says studies show that it works. While scientific, peer-reviewed, double-blind, randomized, large-sample, reproducible studies are an admittedly high standard, they are the gold standard of reliable information. Other literature can run the gamut from a series of case studies that are suggestive of good proof to baseless assertions. Evaluate with care, both what is implied and the actual content of claims.

Some guides suggest countless remedies, while others urge no home homeopathy or other herbal use by lay practitioners due to toxicity risks. Some suggest panaceas and miracle cures. *Cure* is a very strong word.

One book on dog care suggests a cure for osteoarthritis (literally meaning bone-joint inflammation, osteoarthritis is arthritis due to degenerative changes) following a veterinary diagnosis, including a regimen of nutraceuticals (glucosamine, chondroitin, and nutritional enhancers) and herbal supplements (particularly Boswellia, devil's claw root, horsetail, nettle, and yucca), plus therapies such as chiropractic, acupressure, massage, magnetic therapy, or whatever worked best for the animal. The recommendations continue: the temporary use of painkillers such as nonsteroidal anti-inflammatory drugs, regular exercise, avoiding injuries (and quickly attending those that arise), and regularly feeding a superior commercial food or a supplemented home diet at the same time every day. No doubt this program will do a lot to alleviate osteoarthritis (and many other problems as well), but it does not *cure* the disorder.

Other literature complains about the conventional veterinary empire suppressing alternatives. Does the Empire strike backtalk? Certainly there is a spectrum of acceptance, with some vets and other scientists being open-minded while others reject all alternative therapies. Rather than argue how much turf-guarding occurs by the conventional medical establishment, consider those in the alternative treatment field who rail about persecution. It is in the interest of everyone who cares for animals to pursue the best treatments. Be extremely wary of those advocating a therapist or therapy that they claim is persecuted by the Establishment.

Just do that good research before choosing.

The Cat's Meow: Raccoon 1, Kitty 0

Sharkbait hid after the fight. She's a little orange tabby cat with a big voice, long white whiskers, and no reservations about leaping onto unsuspecting peoples' shoulders. The owner guesses it was a raccoon that thoroughly beat up Sharkbait one day. Woods and a pond right outside the house make an inviting setting for wildlife as well as the family with their large assortment of animals.

The owner is a levelheaded woman with considerable skill in handling animals, and not burdened by squeamishness. When she found Sharkbait tucked silently into a corner with his nasty combat wounds, she set to work cleaning up the battered cat.

"I was most worried about abscesses with the punctures," she said.

She flushed and cleaned the wounds on the back of the cat's neck. A fan of natural treatments and a bit reserved about pharmaceutical intervention, she is willing to conflate the two schools of thought: alternative treatments and modern, science-based medicine. She uses arnica creams on sore muscles and doses colds with echinacea and vitamin C.

Healing by third intent (also known as *per tertium intentionem*) is when primary closure of wounds is delayed. Neglected injuries on an animal that is not cared for must heal by third intent, but healing by third intent is not necessarily a matter of neglect. Wounds that were grossly contaminated are often allowed to heal by third intent in order to ensure that some small, missed bit of contamination is not sutured up within a deep wound to later become infected. Sharkbait was monitored for third intent healing.

But Sharkbait was not recovering from the battle.

Although the wounds did not appear to have significant local infection, the cat's condition deteriorated. Sharkbait looked terrible, and wasn't healing or eating. The owner knew she was losing the cat, and she didn't hesitate to get advanced intervention, including a full course of antibiotics.

She snaps her fingers relating the results of injected antibiotic treatment. "Turned right around, right away."

Modern medicine stepped in to save the dying cat. She's back to making noise and mischief, exactly as a cat should, especially one named Sharkbait.

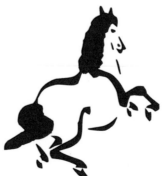

When to Choose Alternative Treatments

WHEN READING AND learning, do not be tempted to administer home health care beyond your capabilities. Lay guides tend to lack good patient-assessment information, nor is it a lay guide's place to teach the reader how to thoroughly give a medical appraisal. Go to a professional for evaluation and discuss all treatment options. If you decide to try a particular treatment, find a good, reputable provider.

A horse with laminitis needs a good veterinarian and farrier. A dog hit by a car or suffering from bloat needs a good veterinary surgeon. Using alternative treatments as primary care for animals with significant illnesses or injuries conflicts with giving the animal the best possible care. Modern medicine gives the best chance to animals with serious and critical conditions. Thus, deciding *when* is actually a bit easier and cleaner than deciding *how* to choose alternative treatments.

Chronic conditions, certain degenerative disorders, and less severe ailments better afford an opportunity to consider alternatives. For anyone interested in trying alternatives in less critical situations, the key remains to explore the alternatives carefully in order to choose the best treatment.

Many people approach alternative treatments with an attitude of *Why not try it?* To each their own, and again, the placebo effect is sometimes quite beneficial. But if the alternative is not shown to work, displaces competent care, or places a financial burden on the owner, then it's a strong argument not to try the alternative. Consider an algorithm approach on making this decision.

Three Steps to Deciding on Alternatives

Determine whether conventional medicine has done all it can for the animal's condition.

Yes, there are some on the fringe who would never see a conventional veterinarian. However, if science-based medicine offers a safe, proven, and effective treatment for the condition, then science-based medicine is the best option. If the outcome from that treatment has a poor prognosis or risks significant side effects, then it is understandable to investigate alternatives.

Determine whether the animal will tolerate the treatment.

Be cautious to weigh the whole scenario when considering a treatment. For example, an animal who does not tolerate travel to and from a practitioner will not receive as great a benefit as an animal who is not bothered by travel, and may actually have his condition worsened by the stress. A treatment is contraindicated if the benefits are outweighed by the negative impacts.

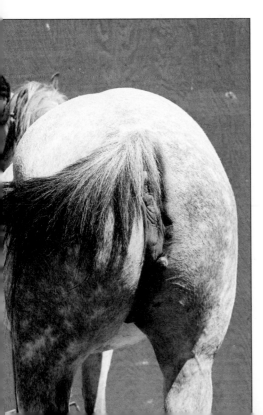

Determine whether there is any potential for harm from the treatment.

Many treatments carry risks of side effects, with varying degrees of how commonly the problems are encountered and varying degrees of severity for those negative outcomes. Use all of your research and resources to get a solid answer to your questions.

LEFT: **Know whether a problem is a reasonable candidate for alternative treatment. This mare's tumor needs conventional care first.**

Choosing Your Alternative Treatment Practitioner

Consumers can ask for referrals from their veterinarians, but they cannot rely on the traditional vets to direct them to quality alternative-care options. In some Australian states, for example, it may not be legal for a veterinarian to refer a client to a nontraditional healer, and in the United Kingdom, veterinarians generally must supervise animal treatment in some fashion. However, the final caveat in choosing alternative treatment is this: *Do not exclude one professional from knowledge of the other.* It's best if all of the professional animal care providers attending a patient are aware of the others' efforts.

Again, selection of a reputable animal care practitioner falls to the consumer.

Reuse the standard research tools of this book—referrals, organizations, libraries, electronic databases, and the Internet—to find practitioners. And then be prepared to ask the prospective practitioners smart questions.

INTERVIEWING PROSPECTIVE PRACTITIONERS

The final step in securing good alternative treatment is locating that good practitioner. Ask good questions in order to get enough information to make a valid assessment of the practitioner's offerings.

- *What percent of their practice is devoted to this treatment?*
- *Where did they get their training?*
- *How long was the training program?*
- *What is the best and worst result that might be achieved?*
- *Would they recommend this treatment for their own animals?*
- *What are all of the risks and benefits?*
- *Ask the hows. How long might it take, how much will it cost, how many successes and failures has the treatment had when done by each practitioner?*

Then carefully evaluate those answers. Are they facts, opinions, or beliefs? Vague responses or unsupported statements deserve more scrutiny. Make a good selection decision by critically studying the therapist in the same manner you studied the therapy. A specialist's sincere belief in the value of the treatment he offers does not make the practice any more effective. The practitioner may be guessing, incorrect, or stating a belief or opinion as fact, when in reality the belief or opinion is unproven, or worse, disproven.

Try to understand the practitioner's goals, methods, and limitations. Remember the specialists who are not adequately trained, thus not legally allowed to assess a specific medical condition, so they coin a virtual synonym, say *knurdles*, and advise they can detect knurdles. When someone advises that X is *like* diabetes or laminitis or any other conventional term, get a good, clear answer on the *difference* between X and the conventional term. If the practitioner can articulate no meaningful difference between the new term and the commonly understood term, then the practitioner is indeed claiming to have diagnosed or treated the actual condition; if this is diabetes or laminitis or another serious condition that the practitioner is not trained to assess and treat, then the practitioner is clearly treading beyond the bounds of his or her education and abilities.

Some practitioners, some patients, and some consumers are more suggestible than others. While generalizations can be made and argued, patients who are more reactive tend to be better candidates for inducing a placebo response. What really counts to an individual is that individual's experience. Make that experience a good one through smart researching.

Admittedly, the studying is more difficult for some. People *more* grounded in science in general—and in medicine in specific—can have greater difficulty with alternative concepts. Some practitioners simply do not use accepted medical terms. For example, they may refer to foods creating moisture or drying dampness in the animal, instead of addressing conditions of edema or dehydration. New terms for not-so-new practices abound. However, when theories, opinions, and hopes are stated as fact, the statement and its speaker are questionable. Certainly, some alternative treatments can become moneymakers for the practitioners who employ them. The wise consumer must try to evaluate the practitioner's motives.

Valid reasons make for valid choices. There is no harm in either a skeptical or an open-minded approach to determining who will be your practitioner. Continue to specifically seek out advice critical of a therapy before engaging in a course of treatment. Pool your resources and tell your veterinarian if you're seeking a nontraditional practitioner. When you've made a selection, share the person's name with the vet. And tell that alternative practitioner about the veterinarian's assessment and treatment of the animal's condition.

Always, always give science a chance, because conventional veterinary experience, diagnostics, and treatment modalities represent an animal's best chance. Examine all the options—there is a tremendous range of choices. Because you are responsible for your animal's health, the *how* and *when* of making the choice for alternative treatment merits thoughtful consideration. Despite anyone's interest in alternative treatments, the best of modern medicine represents an animal's best chance when confronted with a significant illness or injury.

Some vets and other practitioners are skeptics with little or no familiarization training on alternative treatments. Other veterinarians may be quite familiar with dozens of alternatives but reject them all as worthless.

Some practitioners are true believers in a host of alternatives. One veterinarian writes that pet guardians should shoot love at their animals. A small animal veterinary instructor from one of the United States' most prestigious TCVM educational institutions advised that it is possible to briefly detect a horse's pulse by placing one's fingers on the horse's pulse point and simultaneously checking one's own pulse with the other hand because the pulses would switch to the same beat for a short time. (This assertion does not bear out for your author, a paramedic who can palpate pulses on horses when many people must reach for a stethoscope, tested the vet instructor's claim with an assistant who monitored the test horse with a stethoscope. The test horse's heart rate auscultated and palpated at 36 beats per minute while the author's pulse palpated regularly at 80 beats per minute.)

An equine vet asked to evaluate the previous vet's assertion about pulse detection laughed and wondered if the first vet instructor had said anything else that raised the eyebrows. (Well, there was that bit about all females being inherently deficient in their blood and needing to avoid ginseng because of their yang.) The equine vet challenged the author to touch a horse's pulse and have the same beat show up in her wrist. The author was again unable to count a horse's pulse by checking her own.

Other veterinarians are somewhere in the middle of these two ends of the skeptic–true believer spectrum. These tend to be the practitioners who, to some extent, accept the blending of conventional and alternative treatments. It is left to the consumer to study, to choose, to shop with discretion.

The Shopping Trip: Nutrition, Evidence, and Straw

A resplendently happy Labrador hauled his person inside the specialty pet food store, poked the shop cat in the head, and then slurped from the community water bowl in the center of the room.

"He likes our water," the proprietor said. "He really likes our water."

The average Labrador likes water in the way other critters like air, but the store owner assured me this was special water.

What could be so special about the water? I wondered.

"It's filtered."

Indeed, the store staff recommended filtered water for all animals. City water is too treated, they say. Too much chlorine and other chemicals. And water from wells could have groundwater contamination, heavy metals, or unhealthy microbes. The only way to ensure a dog or cat's drinking water is clean and safe is to use filtered water.

Nutrition is the largest block of alternative interest in the pet world. There are now many stores like the one I visited, specializing in companion animal—mostly feline and canine—nutrition.

The staff is generous with their time and experience, their stock of specialty foods and treats is absolutely amazing, and they also offer a number of natural products for various pet afflictions. They moved quickly to help a new customer, an older woman, in for the first time. She wanted to go natural and healthy, keep her cat chemical-free. One store employee showed her kibble intended to help align a cat's meridians.

The customer nodded.

The register rang and rang, and she paid the three-digit bill with her credit card. Her thirteenth bag of food would be free, and the staff told her she would probably reach that free bag in about a year.

Beyond the cat food aisle, I studied the dog foods. Bison snacks. Buffalo treats. Chicken with apricot dinners. Grain-free surf and turf. Organic hearts. Sweet potato and duck meat kibble. Pork and applesauce dog food. Salmon and *hand-picked* vegetables with eggs and cheese for special dogs. The meals are slow-simmered and prepared in small batches.

The store owner talked to the man with the Labrador about optimizing the Lab's health. He was trying to decide between the venison meal and the herring meal.

Appetite percolating, I listened to the owner's pitch. She offered not just the promise of better health for the healthy Labrador, but also the general benefits of natural food, of going chemical-free, and of avoiding larger corporations and recall scandals.

Actually, these prime pet foods experience recalls just like the common kibbles seen in feed stores and veterinary offices. Pet foods that used to be considered premium are now supplanted in the minds of premium-seekers by the trendy companies stocked at the specialty companion animal nutrition store.

One premium brand recalled food in 2010 after discovering one of their supplement premixers left their cat food formula with accidentally incorrect zinc and potassium levels. In another case in the same year, a veterinarian's dog, fed a premium diet, developed signs of hypercalcemia (calcium level in the blood above normal). About three dozen dogs on the same food had the same problem: hypercalcemia secondary to vitamin D toxicosis.

Store staff assured another customer that the big brands experienced these sorts of problems far more than the small premium companies stocked on the shelves. This is a putative belief—it's put forth as true, accepted as true, but based on inconclusive data.

The saleswoman explained to the customer that human-grade manufacturing practices are not required in the United States for pet food manufacturers. She's right. Slaughter animals classified as 4D (dead, dying, diseased, or disabled) are not allowed to be processed for human consumption but may be rendered for pet food.

I studied the supplements and found a common warning on the bottles:

This product has not been evaluated by the U.S. Food and Drug Administration.

This product is not intended to diagnose, treat, cure, or prevent any disease.

Skeptics call these two sentences *the Quack Miranda*. The sentences became legally attached to countless alternative supplements sold in the United States under the mandate of the Dietary Supplement Health and Education Act of 1994.

The DSHE Act (or DSHEA) also required good manufacturing practices (known in the industry as GMP, or CGMP for current good manufacturing practices)—which had long been required for pharmaceuticals, but not for dietary supplements—to finally be required on dietary supplements *for people*. And there's the catch. Regulation over dietary supplements *for animals* is minimal.

Alternative practitioners applauded the passage of the DSHEA as a boon to consumer freedom. Skeptics groaned about how it eroded oversight from the supplement industry.

In another section of the store, I studied the natural pet remedies for sale. There were homeopathic drops for a variety of emotional problems. The packages promised to correct a cat's shyness, alleviate a dog's travel anxiety, and more.

Another flier urged me not to poison my pet with chemicals when there were natural ways to control ticks and fleas.

A 1998 article in the *Journal of Veterinary Diagnostic Investigation* detailed the case of a cat owner who applied Australian tea tree (*Melaleuca alternifolia*) oil as a natural flea repellent. The owner had bought the product from a pet catalog. All three cats were poisoned by the tea tree oil flea treatment, and one died. The cats must have suffered from their owner's well-intentioned effort. Surely the owner suffered as well.

A woman left the store with a small bag of food that cost nearly fifty dollars. I could hear the man waiting for her outside say, "The stuff from Safeway is just as good."

But there *is* a difference in the quality of different pet foods. In the spring of 1998, the FDA surveyed a number of dog foods and found pentobarbital traces in many samples. This is due to the allowed practice of rendering humanely euthanized animals (animals intentionally given a lethal dose of pentobarbital) to be processed into animal food.

I interviewed a number of veterinarians who are strong supporters of evidence-based medicine. These vets regularly publish and speak and blog about the risks associated with not relying on good science and the attendant failures of alternative treatments. We talked about many issues in animal care and alternative treatments, including nutrition.

Animal owners spend greater effort and interest and money on feed than on any other facet of pet care. As the science-based vets point out, there are many myths floating around about nutrition. The alternative world's constant push of what is natural can be at odds with sense—what a wolf or bobcat eats in the wild is of course not the same as what the average dog or cat is fed. However, nor is the diet of a captive wolf or cougar the same as what it would eat in the wild. Also, captive predators like wolves and cougars generally live much longer than their wild counterparts, and diet can play a role in that longevity.

We reviewed the vignettes of real experiences of alternative treatments. We couldn't find one that could be shown to have worked—such is the standing dichotomy of alternatives. If an alternative treatment could be scientifically shown to work, it would not be an alternative—it would instead be mainstream, science-based medicine.

"It's like fuzzy dice in your car," one vet told me.

Fuzzy dice?

His analogy compared care of an animal to a vehicle. The vehicle has to have certain care and maintenance, must have fuel and oil. People do things to their cars—dangle fuzzy dice from the rearview mirror—that are unnecessary but the owners feel good doing it.

This vet was tired of alternative proponents mischaracterizing science-based vets as being anti-alternatives. "We're not," he said. "We're *for* anything that works. If it's shown to work, to help animals, we'll use it. If a treatment is not shown to work, we won't use it."

Certainly, science-based vets—and the majority of veterinarians are science-based—are the targets of a great deal of name-calling by many proponents of alternative treatments.

They're in the pocket of big corporations, of Big Pharma; they're just in it for the money.

They're not. They're in the field of animal medicine due to a sincere interest in caring for animals.

Straw-man arguments—in which one contests not the issue specifically raised but instead argues a different point, such as attacking the person making the statement—frequently arise in the debate between alternative treatments and evidence-based medicine. Alternative advocates cannot win a science-based review.

Remember the cyborg horse? Refer now to the photograph of the gray mare with the growth on her haunch. That growth simply fell off one day. Might the growth on the cyborg gelding's eye similarly have resolved spontaneously, with no intervention? In other words, might the cyborg gelding have healed himself without the alternative veterinarian's special salve, just like the gray mare did?

Among the other real-life examples, again, no proof can be demonstrated: the dog with lick granuloma, whose owners were so pleased that the dog stopped licking and let his wounds heal after acupuncture, the horse believed to have ulcers that were believed to have been healed or prevented with a homeopathic remedy, the parrot with a crystal in his water, the psychic. Not one alternative treatment can be scientifically shown to have worked, but certain experiences did stun some of my science-based review vets.

"A psychic? You talked to a psychic!"

Well, yes, because I was interested in hearing what she'd say, and paying the price of admission is the way to see the show.

He was frustrated. "Would you actually talk to a psychic when you really needed help with a critical problem?"

It's not likely, but it's possible, and I said that he'd do the same. That stopped him.

I told him when he'd do it. "Imagine your child didn't come home from school. No leads. Everyone's checked everything. Your kid is gone. It's been a week. It's been a month. Some friend brings a psychic in. All you have to do is talk to the psychic."

"I'd do it. Of course. But that's just grasping at straws."

We talked about straws, about hope and faith and good intentions, and the difference between knowledge and belief. Ultimately, that difference is the gap between modern medicine and alternative treatments.

The field of alternative treatments for animals is not a case of *you're either with us or against us.* There is room for disagreement, room for diverse belief systems. There is room for reasonable respect as well.

No one gets to demand that another person fit into one dichotomy. While we may want to make someone disagree or agree, the person could opt out of the discussion, find the challenge to be the wrong challenge.

Alternative treatments for animals are here to stay.

Point and Counterpoint: Nutritionists and Tradition v. Hard Science and Dead Ponies

HORSES FREQUENTLY INGEST small amounts of dirt and sand as they naturally forage on grasses. In modern horse-keeping, horses are often confined on bare dirt, which exposes them to even greater opportunities to regularly ingest excess amounts of dirt and sand. Accumulated sand in a horse's intestine may be visible on a radiograph or audible through a stethoscope.

When horses suffer from an episode of significant gastrointestinal distress (colic), the cause is sometimes believed to be due to the ingestion of excess sand, and termed *sand colic*.

Both well-established traditional care for horses and modern equine nutritionists often recommend the same very well-accepted preventative treatment for sand colic—oral administration of psyllium to help the horse clear the sand from his colon, thus relieving the pain and dysfunction.

Psyllium, also called ispaghula, is composed of the seeds and seed husks of an Indian herb called *Plantago ovata*; it is very high in water-soluble fiber that forms a gel-like substance with liquids, thus it is used as an over-the-counter treatment for constipation in humans. Metamucil is one common brand name of psyllium intended for humans.

People have interpolated their treatment for their problems to their horses. However, without scientific backing, interpolations are suspect. Unlike humans, horses intake tremendous amounts of fiber in their natural diet. Does it really make sense that a fiber supplement would help an average horse with gastro-intestinal difficulty?

Finally, two small, well-designed studies have examined the efficacy of removing sand from the equine gastrointestinal tract via the administration of psyllium.

In the first study, sand was placed into the test horses' stomachs via nasogastric tube (a tube inserted through the nostril into the stomach). Some of these test horses were then given psyllium and some were not treated. The welfare of all horses in the study was carefully monitored and their feces were examined to determine how well the psyllium had aided in the excretion of sand from the horses' gastrointestinal tracts. In this study, the administration of psyllium had no bearing on the horses' natural ability to excrete sand.

In a study of ponies who were already scheduled for euthanasia, sand was surgically placed into the ponies' cecums (part of the equine hindgut, or lower gastrointestinal tract). Some of the ponies were treated with psyllium, and all were monitored for sand excretion in their feces. Again, the administration of psyllium had no significant bearing on how well the ponies guts removed the sand.

The conclusion is that some equines remove sand from their guts better than others, but the administration of psyllium—long believed by traditionists and modern nutritionists to help horses with the removal of sand—does not appear to help at all.

The best treatment for sand colic is prevention by minimizing opportunities for the horses to eat their forage directly from a dirt surface.

These two studies highlight the need for scientific research to illuminate well-accepted practices. Both modern alternative nutritionists and traditional horse-keeping practices that would not have been considered under the alternative umbrella have long advocated supplementing or treating sand colic with psyllium, yet the science shows that the treatment is ineffective. It is important to discern the difference between what we think we know and what we actually know when we evaluate treatments.

Integration

TODAY'S CHOICE IS frequently an integrative blending of conventional and alternative treatments. Yet some consumers may lean heavily toward alternatives. For those who find appeal in bucking the Establishment for the sake of it, recognize that anyone can hang a shingle or self-proclaim an expertise that is patently false even though the practitioner might truly believe his or her own claims.

Other consumers may lean heavily away from alternatives. For those who twitch when hearing broad unsupported statements, who don't want to wear a toga while chanting and sniffing incense over good dogs, cats, and horses, consider the potential benefits of holistic care, strongly emphasizing an animal's physical and mental health, maintaining a healthy diet and exercise regimen.

Good modern medicine—whether it is called allopathic, traditional, mainstream, evidence-based, scientific, biomedicine, orthodox, or conventional medicine—is perhaps one hundred years old, but it is indeed very, very good. The safest and smartest choice for those who choose alternative treatments for their animals is to integrate the carefully chosen alternative with solid conventional care.

Remember the guinea-pig dog with hip dysplasia? Whether his condition was due to bone changes, joint laxity, or deficient kidney jing, we never did find an alternative practitioner who simply wanted him exercised more. While the conventional veterinarian who diagnosed hip dysplasia would give the same diagnosis with the accurate or phony history, because he made his diagnosis with radiographs on an anesthetized dog, no alternative practitioner ever asserted a different diagnosis when presented with a large, sore-hipped shepherd.

Exploring alternative treatments for animals is best done with intelligence, curiosity, and responsibility. The work of choosing comes before the choice. While the heavy exploration required of the consumer is a large burden, so is giving good care to an animal. Remember that the *how* phase, done well, enables the *when* of choosing alternative treatment to be fairly straightforward.

Readers are again urged to be cautious consumers of alternative treatments and to never risk an animal's health by denying their animals competent, conventional care. If you wish to explore alternatives, integrating conventional and alternative care is the smart way to ensure your animal receives the best care. The standing dichotomy of alternatives remains that if they were conclusively, scientifically proven to be of demonstrable benefit, then they would not be alternatives—they would be mainstream medicine.

There is value to be found among many alternative therapies and therapists, and there is a great deal of nonsense as well.

Again, selection of a reputable animal care practitioner falls to the consumer. Are there red flags that should warn us away from an alternative treatment or practitioner? Yes.

THINK VERY CAREFULLY ABOUT TREATMENTS
- *that rely entirely on anecdotes or testimonials for support;*
- *with undisclosed, proprietary, or secret ingredients;*
- *advertised with highly alarmist claims about the malady to be treated;*
- *promoted with extraordinary praise, such as "miraculous"; or*
- *with little information available even after a careful search.*

AND BE VERY WARY OF ANY PRACTITIONER WHO
- *is overtly hostile toward established medicine;*
- *is reluctant to disclose his or her education and experience;*
- *hawks his or her treatment as the very best available;*
- *suggests delaying necessary veterinary care for your animal; or*
- *claims an extraordinarily high success rate.*

With the above caveats, always be cautious of therapies that have little sensible, reasonable information available. Understood in this warning is that you *are* going to seek whatever information is available, reading both the pros and cons. Check referrals of the therapists and consult with a competent veterinarian as you, the smart consumer, go about exploring alternative treatments for your animal.

For those who reject all alternative treatments because they have not been scientifically proven, remember what also cannot be proven: your love for an animal and an animal's love for you.

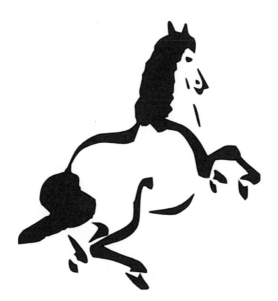

Resources

Organizations and Websites

ANIMAL CARE/PRIMARY VETERINARY ORGANIZATIONS

American Veterinary Medical Association
1931 North Meacham Road
Suite 100
Schaumburg, IL 60173
(847) 925-8070
Fax (847) 925-1329
avmainfo@avma.org
www.avma.org
Founded in 1863. Member organization of over 75,000 veterinarians, mission is to improve animal health and advance the veterinary profession.

Australian Veterinary Association
Unit 40, 2a Herbert Street
St Leonards NSW 2065
www.ava.com.au

British Veterinary Association
7 Mansfield Street
London
W1G 9NQ
+44(0)20 7636 6541
Fax +44(0)20 7436 2970
bvaq@bva.co.uk
www.bva.co.uk
Member organization of 11,000 promoting the veterinary profession. Weekly journal.

Canadian Veterinary Medical Association
339 Booth Street
Ottawa, ON
K1R 7K1
(613) 236-1162
Fax (613) 236-9681
admin@cvma-acmv.org
www.canadianveterinarians.net

New Zealand Veterinary Association
PO Box 11-212
Wellington, New Zealand
nzva@vets.org.nz
www.vets.org.nz

Veterinary Ireland
13 The Courtyard Kilcarbery Park
Nangor Road
Dublin 22
HQ@vetireland.ie
www.veterinary-ireland.org

World Veterinary Association
www.worldvet.org
International collection of veterinary associations.

⁂

Anti–Health Fraud

The Australian Council Against Health Fraud
www.acahf.org.au

www.quackwatch.org
Site dedicated to reviewing alternative treatments and exposing
   questionable practices.

www.veterinarywatch.org
Site dedicated to reviewing alternative veterinary treatments and
   questionable practices.

www.vet-task-force.com
Veterinary Task Force with a special review of Alternative Medicine.

❦

Acupuncture

American Academy of Veterinary Acupuncture
100 Roscommon Drive
Suite 320
Middletown, CT 06457-1591
(860) 635-6400
Fax (860) 635-6400
www.aava.org
Founded in 1998. Member organization, affiliated with the
   International Veterinary Acupuncture Society, promoting veteri-
   nary acupuncture and TCVM.

International Veterinary Acupuncture Society
P.O. Box 271395
Fort Collins, CO 80527
(970) 266-0666
Fax (970) 266-0777
Ivasoffice@aol.com
www.ivas.org
Founder David H. Jaggar, D.C., MRCVS

Bach Flower Remedies

Bach Centre
Mount Vernon, Bakers Lane
Brightwell-cum-Sotwell
Oxon OX10 0PZ
U.K.

+44 (0) 1491 834678

www.bachcentre.com

Botanicals

The New Zealand Association of Medical Herbalists

P.O. Box 12582, Hamilton, NZ

www.nzamh.org

Veterinary Botanical Medicine Association

Jasmine C. Lyon, Executive Director

1785 Poplar Dr.

Kennesaw, GA 30144

office@vbma.org

www.vbma.org

Bowen Technique

www.bowendirectory.com

Referral and informational website on the Bowen technique

Chiropractic

American Veterinary Chiropractic Association

442154 East 140 Road

Bluejacket, OK 74333

(918) 784-2231

Fax (918) 784-2675

avcainfo@junct.com

www.animalchiropractic.org

Founded in 1989. Membership organization,
  has an accreditation commission.

Maintains a referral list:

www.avcadoctors.com

Australian equine chiropractor referral list
www.horsedirectory.com.au/qld/health_service/
chiropractor/index.html

McTimoney College of Chiropractic
Kimber House
1 Kimber Road
Abingdon
Oxfordshire
OXI4 IBZ
chiropractic@mctimoney-college.ac.uk
www.mctimoney-college.ac.uk
Options for Animals
Wellsville, KS 66092
(309) 658-2920
Fax (309) 658-2622
www.animalchiro.com
Established 1988.

The Oxford College of Equine Physical Therapy
mctimoney-corley.com

Homeopathy

The Academy of Veterinary Homeopathy
P. O. Box 9280
Wilmington, DE 19809
(866) 652-1590
www.theavh.org
Founded in 1995, has a referral list.

British Association of Homeopathic Veterinary Surgeons
www.bahvs.com
Formed in 1982, Membership organization of about 140 meant to
increase professional awareness and encourage homeopathic
training for veterinarians. Holds an annual congress, publishes
quarterly newsletters, and maintains a referral list.

The Faculty of Homeopathy
Hahnemann House
29 Park Street West
Luton, Beds
LU1 3BE
United Kingdom
Provides education in homeopathy to certified veterinarians.

International Association for Veterinary Homeopathy
Sonnhaldstr. 18
CH-8370 Sirnach
Switzerland

Holistic Animal Groups

American Holistic Veterinary Medical Association
Carvel G. Tiekert, Executive Director
2218 Old Emmorton Road
Bel Air, MD 21015
(410) 569-0795
Fax (410) 569-2346
office@ahvma.org
www.ahvma.org
Incorporated 1985. Member organization, publishes a journal, gives
    seminars and holds an annual conference. Has a practitioner list:
www.holisticvetlist.com
http://www.naturalholistic.com/referral.htm

Holistic Animal Therapy Association of Australia, Inc.
P.O. Box 513
Grafton, NSW. 2460
Australia
office@hataa.asn.au
www.hataa.asn.au
Formed 1998. Publishes newsletter and maintains a referral list.

International Alliance for Animal Therapy and Healing
www.iaath.com

Hydrotherapy

To locate an animal swimming pool in the U.K., visit this site:
http://www.natural-animal-health.co.uk/find-therapist.htm
Association of Canine Water Therapy
325 E. Washington Street #237
Sequim, WA 98382
www.caninewatertherapy.com

Kinesiology

International College of Applied Kinesiology
www.icak.com

Massage

Association of Chartered Physiotherapists in Animal Therapy
British organization of animal physical therapists who work on the
    basis of referrals from veterinarians.
www.acpat.org

International Association of Animal Massage and Bodywork
Organization of fifteen U.S. and Canadian member schools
www.IAAMB.org

International Equine Body Worker Association
www.iebwa.com

Nambudripad's Allergy Elimination Technique for animals

(Veterinary NAET)
www.vetnaet.com/referral.html

Naturopathy

American Veterinary Naturopathy Association
P. O. Box 243

Sargent, GA 30275

(206) 350-2862

info@avna.us

www.avna.us

Founded 2005. Accredits a few veterinary naturopathy schools.

To locate naturopathic vets in Australia and New Zealand, check this site:

http://www.usenature.com/petcare.htm

Rolfing

www.equinesi.com

Equine Structural Integration site

In Australia, referrals may be received by calling

61-2-9122 6770

info@rolfing.org.au

www.rolfing.org.au/horse_rolfing.htm

Scenar

ISTA International SCENAR Technology Association

Bulgarian-initiated SCENAR group with members in twenty nations, focused on human therapeutic applications.

www.scenartech.com

TCVM

The Chi Institute

9700 West Hwy 318

Reddick, FL 32686

www.chi-institute.com

www.tcvm.com

admin@tcvm.com

(800) 891-1986

(352) 591-5385

Fax (866) 700-8772

(352) 591-2854

Founded in 1998. Private school teaching beginning and advanced courses in TCVM to vets and vet techs. Hundreds of graduates, has referral list.

Healing Oasis Wellness Center
2555 Wisconsin Street
Sturtevant, WI 53177
(262) 884-9549
(262) 886-6460
www.thehealingoasis.com
Teaches veterinary Chinese herbology.
Referral list: http://www.thehealingoasis.com/html/doctors_that_completed_program.html
Healing Oasis Wellness Centre of Canada
www.veterinarychiropractic.ca

New Mexico Chinese Herbal Veterinary Medicine Course
1925 Juan Tabo NE Ste E
Albuquerque, NM 87112
505-450-4325
FAX: 505-332-4775
also listed at:
2237 West Schaumburg Road
Schaumburg, IL 60194
(847) 710-4325
Fax (847) 891-9040

Therapeutic Touch

www.therapeutic-touch.org

TTouch

Linda Tellington-Jones
PO Box 3793
Santa Fe, NM 87501

(866)4-Ttouch [(866) 488-6824]

(505) 455-2945

info@Ttouch.com

www.tteam-ttouch.com

Practitioner directory:

http://tteam-ttouch.com/pracDirectory.shtml

Tuning Fork Therapy

Kairos Institute of Sound Healing

157 Pacheco Road

Box 8

Llano de San Juan, NM 87543

(505) 587-2689

Fax (505) 587-0514

info@acutonics.com

www.acutonics.com

Teaches Acutonics, the use of tuning forks applied to acupuncture
points; believes the therapy stimulates and balances the body's
energy fields. Does not specifically advocate the use on dogs, however veterinary and animal chiropractic practitioners sometimes
use tuning forks.

Veterinary Orthopedic Manipulation

www.vomtech.com

❧❦

Additional Resources

www.altvetmed.com
Compendium site of alternative veterinary treatments.

www.fda.gov/AnimalVeterinary/default.htm
U.S. Food and Drug Administration's Veterinary section.

www.ncbi.nlm.nih.gov/entrez/query.fcgi?CMD=search&DB=pubmed
CAM articles on PubMed. Free searches.

www.drspinello.com/altmed/acuvet/acuvet.swf
Link to Imrie, et al, presentation on acupuncture and TCM/TCVM.

European Medicines Agency
7 Westferry Circus
Canary Wharf
London E14 4HB
United Kingdom
www.emea.europa.eu
Similar to the U.S. FDA, regulating human and veterinary medicines.

Foundation for Integrative Health
12 Chillingworth Road
London N78QJ
United Kingdom
www.fih.org.uk
Foundation promoting human complementary medicine.

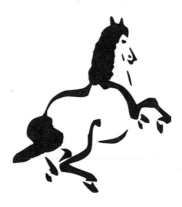

References

Andrews, Ted *How to Heal with Color* Llewellyn: St. Paul, MN, 1992.

Arora, David *All That the Rain Promises, and More . . .* Ten Speed Press: Berkeley, 1991.

Alternative Medicine: The Definitive Guide, second edition, Larry Trivieri and John W. Anderson, eds. Celestial Arts: Berkeley, 2002.

Aschwanden, Christie *Good to Go: What the Athlete in All of Us Can Learn from the Strange Science of Recovery* W.W. Norton: New York, 2019.

Ballner, Maryjean *Dog Massage* St. Martin's Griffin: New York, 2001.

Beale, Brian, DVM and Brenda Adderly, MHA. *The Arthritis Cure for Pets* Little, Brown and Company: Boston, 2000.

Bean-Raymond, Denise *Illustrated Guide to Holistic Care for Horses* Quarry: Beverley, MA, 2009.

Berger, J. N., S. J. Spier, R. Davies, I. A. Gardner, C. M. Leutenegger, M. Bain. Behavioral and physiological responses of weaned foals treated with equine appeasing pheromone: A double-blind, placebo-controlled, randomized trial. *J Vet Behvr* (2013) 8, 265–277.

Bird, Catherine *A Healthy Horse the Natural Way: The Horse Owner's Guide to Using Herbs, Massage, Homeopathy and Other Natural Therapies* Lyons Press: Guilford, CT, 2006.

Brennan, Mary L., DVM with Norma Eckroate *Complete Holistic Care and Healing for Horses* Trafalgar: North Pomfret, VT, 2001.

Bromiley, Mary *Natural Methods for Equine Health* Blackwell Science: London, 1994.

Burger, Sandra *Horse Owner's Field Guide to Toxic Plants* Breakthrough: Ossining, NY, 1996.

Burroughs, Stanley *Healing for the Age of Enlightenment Balanced Nutrition Vita Flex Color Therapy* 1976; renewed 1993 by Alisa Burroughs.

Cambridge Illustrated History of Medicine Roy Porter, editor Cambridge University Press: Cambridge and New York, 1996.

Carlson, Delbert G., DVM, and James M. Griffin, MD *Dog Owner's Home Veterinary Handbook* Howell: New York, 1980.

Cassileth, Barrie, PhD. *The Alternative Medicine Handbook: The Complete Reference Guide to Alternative and Complimentary Therapies* Norton: New York, 1998.

Coates, Margrit *Healing for Pets: The Animal Lover's Essential Guide to Using Healing Energy* Random House: London, 2003.

Coates, Margrit *Hands-On Healing for Horses: The Essential Guide to Using Hands-On Healing Energy with Horses* Sterling Publishing; New York, 2002.

Coleby, Pat *Natural Horse Care* Acres USA: Austin, TX, 2001.

Collinge, William, MPH, PhD. *The American Holistic Health Association Complete Guide to Alternative Medicine* Warner: New York, 1996.

Conti, L. M. C., T. Champion, U. C. Guberman, C. H. T. Mathias, S. L. Fernandes, E. G. M. Silva, M. A. Lazaro, A. D. C. G. Lopes, V. R. Fortunato. Evaluation of environment and a feline facial pheromone analogue on physiological and behavioral measures in cats. *J Fel Med Surg*. Dec. 10, 2015.

De Baïracli Levy, Juliette *The Complete Herbal Handbook for the Dog and Cat* Faber and Faber: London, 1992.

Denoix, Jean-Marie, and Jean-Pierre Pailloux *Physical Therapy and Massage for the Horse* Trafalgar Square Publishing: North Pomfret, VT, 2005.

Dodds, W. Jean, Laverdue, Diana R. *Canine Nutrigenomics: The Science of Feeding Your Dog for Optimal Health*. Dogwise EBooks, 2017.

Dorland's Illustrated Medical Dictionary 31st edition, Saunders: Philadelphia, 2007.

Douglass, William Campbell, MD. *Hydrogen Peroxide: Medical Miracle* Second Opinion Publishing: Atlanta, GA, 1995.

Eckstein, Warren, with Denise Madden *Memoirs of a Pet Therapist* Ballantine: New York, 1998.

Eden, Donna *Energy Medicine: Balance Your Body's Energies for Optimum Health, Joy and Vitality* Putnam: New York, 1998.

Editors of *Pets Speak* Rodale: Emmaus, PA, 2000.

Elsbeth, Marguerite *Crystal Medicine* Llewellyn: St. Paul, MN, 1997.

Falewee, C., E. Gaultier, C. Lafont, L. Bougrat, P. Pageat. Effect of a synthetic equine maternal pheromone during a controlled fear-eliciting situation. *App An Behvr Sci*, Elsevier, Jan. 25, 2006.

Fogle, Bruce, Dr., *Natural Dog Care* DK Publishing: New York, 1999.

Fougère, Barbara, BVSc *The Pet Lover's Guide to Natural Healing for Cats and Dogs* Elsevier Saunders: St. Louis, 2006.

Fox, Michael W., Dr., *The Healing Touch* New Market Press: New York, 1990.

Fugh-Berman, Adriane, MD. *Alternative Medicine: What Works* Williams & Wilkins: Baltimore, 1997.

Fulton, Elizabeth, and Kathleen Prasad *Animal Reiki: Using Energy to Heal the Animals in Your Life* Ulysses Press: Berkeley, 2006.

Gamble, L.-J., J. M. Boesch, C. W. Frye, W. S. Schwark, S. Mann, L. Wolfe, H. Brown, E. S. Berthelsen, and J. J. Wakshlag (2018) "Pharmacokinetics, Safety, and Clinical Efficacy of Cannabidiol

Treatment in Osteoarthritic Dogs." *Front. Vet. Sci.* 5:165. doi: 10.3389/fvets.2018.00165.

Giacomini, Jean-Philippe. Personal communication. July 15, 2019.

Gore, Thomas, DVM, Paula Gore, MT, ASCP BB, and James M. Giffin, MD *Horse Owners Veterinary Handbook* Howell: Hoboken, NJ, 2008.

Guest, D. J., M. R. Smith, and W. R. Allen Equine embryonic stem-like cells and mesenchymal stromal cells have different survival rates and migration patterns following their injection into damaged superficial digital flexor tendon. *Equine Vet* J October 2010, 42(7):636–42.

Heinerman, John, VMD *Natural Pet Cures* Prentice Hall: Paramus, NJ, 1998.

Hoffman, Matthew, ed. *The Doctors Book of Home Remedies for Dogs and Cats* Rodale Press: Emmaus, PA, 1996.

Holloway, Sage *Animal Healing and Vibrational Medicine* Blue Dolphin Publishing: Nevada City, CA, 2001.

Hunter, Francis, MRCVS, VetMF Hom *Homeopathic First Aid Treatment for Pets* Thorsons: London, 1984.

Jacobs, Jennifer *Do You Really Need That Pill?* Skyhorse Publishing: New York, 2018.

Kamen, Daniel *The Well Adjusted Cat: Feline Chiropractic Methods You Can Do* Brookline Books: Cambridge, MA, 1997.

Kamen, Daniel *The Well Adjusted Dog: Canine Chiropractic Methods You Can Do* Brookline Books: Cambridge, MA, 1997.

Kamen, Daniel *The Well Adjusted Horse: Equine Chiropractic Methods You Can Do* Brookline Books: Cambridge, MA, 1999.

Kaptchuk, Ted *The Web That Has No Weaver* McGraw-Hill: New York, 2000.

Kellon, Eleanor M., DVM *Equine Supplements and Nutraceuticals: A Guide to Peak Health and Performance Through Nutrition* Breakthrough Publications: Ossining, NY, 1998.

Kinkade, Amelia *Straight from the Horse's Mouth: How to Talk to Animals and Get Answers* Crown: New York, 2001.

Kligler, Benjamin, and Roberta Anne Lee *Integrative Medicine* McGraw-Hill Professional: New York, 2004.

Krieger, Dolores, PhD, RN. *Therapeutic Touch Inner Workbook* Bear & Company Publishing: Santa Fe, NM, 1997.

Lawrence, Ron, MD, PhD. Paul J. Rosch, MD, FACP, and Judith Plowden *Magnet Therapy: The Pain Cure Alternative* Prima Health: Rocklin, CA, 1998.

Lewin, Rachel *Holistic Healing: A Practical Guide* Astrolog Publishing House: Israel, 1998.

Lidwell, William *How Colors Affect You: What Science Reveals* The Great Courses: Chantilly, VA, 2013.

Lilian, C. De S. O. Batista, Yara P CID, Ana Paula De Almedia, Edlene R. Prudencio *In vitro efficacy of essential oils and extracts of Shinus molle L. against Ctenocephalides felis felis. Parasitology* 143(5):627–638.

Loeb, Jo, and Paul Loeb *Good Dog!* Putnam: New York, 1984.

Malle, Betttina, and Helge Schmikl *The Essential Oil Maker's Handbook* Spikehorn Press: Austin, 2015.

Markoski, M. M. Advances in the use of stem cells in veterinary medicine: from basic research to clinical practice. *Scientifica* (Cairo) June 9, 2016.

Martin, Ann N. *Protect Your Pet* New Sage Press: Troutdale, OR, 2001.

Maughan, R. J., and S. P. Evans Effects of pollen extract upon adolescent swimmers. *Br J Sports Med*. 1982 Se;16(3):142–5.

McCarney, R., P. Fisher, F. Spink, C. Flint, and R. van Haselen Can homeopaths detect homeopathic medicines by dowsing? A randomized double-blind, placebo-controlled trial. *J R Soc Med* 95(4):189–91.

McDonnell, S. M., J. Miller, and W. Vaala. Calming benefit of short-term alpha-casozepine supplements during acclimation to domestic environment and basic ground training of semi-feral ponies. *J Eq Vet Sci* (2012):1–6.

McGinnis, Terri, DVM *The Well Dog Book* Random House: New York, 1991.

Meagher, Jack *Beating Muscle Injuries for Horses* Hamilton: Hamilton, MA, 1985.

Morrison, Scott. Personal communication. June 22, 2019.

Mowrey, Daniel B., PhD. *The Scientific Validation of Herbal Medicine* Cormorant Books: Toronto, 1986.

Nadzan, Danika *How to Be a Dog Psychic* Fairwinds Press: Gloucester, MA, 2005.

Nakaya, Shannon Fujimoto, DVM *Kindred Spirit, Kindred Care* New World Library: Novato, CA, 2005.

Nutrigenetic Testing: Tests Purchased from Four Websites Mislead Consumers. *GAO Highlights* 06-977T, July 27, 2006.

Osweiler, Gary D. *Toxicology* Williams & Wilkins: Media, PA, 1996.

Pascucci, James Vincent, *Equine Structural Integration: Myofascial Release Manual* Sane Systems: United States, 2007.

PDR for Herbal Medicines, third edition, Medical Economics and Physician's Desk Reference -Thomson Healthcare: Montvale, NJ, 2004.

Pitcairn, Richard H., DVM, PhD, and Susan Hubble Pitcairn *Dr. Pitcairn's Complete Guide to Natural Health for Dogs and Cats* Rodale: Emmaus, PA, 1982.

Porter, Mimi *The New Equine Sports Therapy* Bloodhorse, Inc: Lexington, 1998.

Porter, Roy *The Greatest Benefit to Mankind: A Medical History of Humanity* Harper Collins: New York, 1997.

Preston, Lisa *The Ultimate Guide to Horse Feed, Supplements and Nutrition* Skyhorse Publishing: New York, 2016.

Price, Catherine *Vitamania: Our Obsessive Quest for Nutritional Perfection* Penguin Press: New York, 2015.

Puotinen, C. J. *The Encyclopedia of Natural Pet Care* Keats Publishing: Los Angeles, 2000.

Puotinen, C. J. *Natural Remedies for Dogs and Cats* Keats Publishing: Lincolnwood, IL, 1999.

Ramey, David W. *Medications and Supplements for the Horse* Howell: New York, 1996.

Ramey, David W., and Bernard E. Rollin *Complementary and Alternative Veterinary Medicine Considered* Iowa State Press: Ames, Iowa, 2004.

Riotte, Louise *Raising Animals by the Moon: Practical Advice on Breeding, Birthing, Weaning and Raising Animals in Harmony with Nature* Storey Publishing: North Adams, MA, 1999.

Robins, Natalie *Copeland's Cure Homeopathy and the War Between Conventional and Alternative Medicine* Knopf: New York 2005.

Root-Bernstein, Robert, and Michele *Honey, Mud, Maggots and Other Medical Marvels: The Science Behind Folk Remedies and Old Wives' Tales* Houghton Mifflin: Boston, 1997.

Rosenfeld, Isadore *Dr. Rosenfeld's Guide to Alternative Medicine* Random House: New York, 1996.

Schnaubelt, Kurt *Advanced Aromatherapy The Sccience of Essential Oil Therapy* Healing Arts Press; Rochester, VT, 1998.

Schnaubelt, Kurt *The Healing Intelligence of Essential Oils The Science of Advanced Aromatherapy* Healing Arts Press: Rochester, VT, 2011.

Schoen, Allen M., DVM, and Pam Proctor *Love, Miracles, and Animal Healing* Simon & Schuster: New York, 1995.

Schwartz, Cheryl, DVM *Four Paws, Five Directions: A Guide to Chinese Medicine for Cats and Dogs* Celestial Arts: Berkeley, 1996.

Shapiro, Nina *Hype: A Doctor's Guide to Medical Myths, Exaggerated Claims, and Bad Advice—How to Tell What's Real and What's Not* St. Martin's: New York, 2018.

Sherman, R. A., S. Morrison, and D. Ng Maggot Debridement Therapy—A survey of practitioners. *Veterinary Journal* 174(1):86–91.

Shojai, Amy D., and editors of *Prevention for Pets New Choices in Natural Healing for Dogs and Cats* Rodale Press: Emmaus, PA 1999.

Snader, Meredith L., VMD, Sharon L. Willoughby, DVM, Deva Kaur Khalsa, VMD, Craig Denega, BA, and Ihor John Basko, DVM *Healing Your Horse Alternative Therapies* Howell: New York, 1993.

Snow, Amy *The Well-Connected Dog: A Guide to Canine Acupressure* Tallgrass Publishers: Larkspur, CO, 1999.

Somerville, Robert, ed. *The Alternative Advisor: The Complete Guide to Natural Therapies and Alternative Treatments* Time-Life Books: Alexandria, VA, 1997.

Speight, Phyllis *A Study Course in Homeopathy* Health Science Press: Essex, 1979.

Stalker, Douglas, and Clark Glymour, eds. *Examining Holistic Medicine* Prometheus Books: Buffalo, 1985.

Still, J. A clinical study of auriculotherapy in canine thoracolubar disc disease. *JS Afr Vet Assoc.* September 1990, 61(3):102–5.

Sutton, Amanda *The Injury-Free Horse Hands-On Methods for Maintaining Soundness and Health* Trafalgar Square Publishing: North Pomfret, VT, 2001.

Tellington-Jones, Linda, and Sybil Taylor *Getting in TTouch: Understand and Influence Your Horse's Personality* Trafalgar: North Pomfret, VT, 1995.

Tellington-Jones, Linda, and Sybil Taylor *The Tellington TTouch* Penguin: New York, 1992.

Teut, M., R. Lüdke, and A. Warning Reliability of Enderlein's dark-field analysis of live blood. *Altern Ther Health Med* July–August 2006, 12(4):36–41.

Volhard, W., and K. L. Brown *Holistic Guide for a Healthy Dog* Howell Book House: Hoboken, NJ, 2000.

Walker, Kaetheryn *Homeopathic First Aid for Animals: Tales and Techniques from a Country Practitioner* Healing Arts Press: Rochester, VT, 1998.

Wulf-Tilford, Mary L., and Gregory L. Tilford *All You Ever Wanted to Know About Herbs for Pets* Bow Tie Press: Irvine, CA, 1999.

Yarnall, Celeste *Natural Dog Care: A Complete Guide to Holistic Health Care for Dogs* Journey Editions: Boston, 1998.

Zidonis, Nancy A. *Acu-Cat: A Guide to Feline Acupressure* Tallgrass Publishers: Denver, 2000.

Zidonis, Nancy A. *Equine Acupressure: A Working Manual* Tallgrass Publishers: Larkspur, CO, 1999.

Zixin, Lin, Yu Li, Guo Zhengyi, Shen Zhenyu, Zhang Honglin, and Zhang Tongling *Qigong Chinese Medicine or Pseudoscience* Prometheus Books: Amherst, NY, 2000.

Index

About the Author

LISA PRESTON graduated from Oregon Health Science University's Advanced Paramedic Training program in 1984 and later earned a bachelor of science in occupational education, a bachelor of fine arts in languages, and a master's in organizational management. After a career in paramedicine, she worked for many years as an investigator. She has tried or observed many of the alternative treatments in *Alternative Treatments for Animals* and studied them all.

She is a life member of the USDF, the USEA, the USEF, and the Ride and Tie Association.

Find out more at www.lisapreston.com.

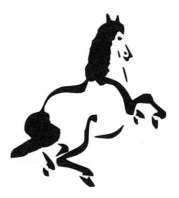